THEY STILL CALL ME DOCTOR

MY LIFE WITH MULTIPLE SCLEROSIS...
A PHYSICIAN'S JOURNEY WITH MS

BARBARA HENICK BACHOW, M. D.

Fulton Books
Meadville, PA

Published by Fulton Books 2024

ISBN 979-8-88982-395-7 (paperback)
ISBN 979-8-88982-973-7 (hardcover)
ISBN 979-8-88982-396-4 (digital)

Printed in the United States of America

am a doctor. I was granted my doctor of medicine degree (MD) in 1979 by the University of Massachusetts, and I did my post-doctoral residencies (in Internal Medicine, followed by Diagnostic Radiology) at major teaching hospitals affiliated with well-known medical schools in Boston. Toward the end of my second residency, I married another physician, and a few months after being granted certification by the American Board of Radiology, I gave birth to our first child. Shortly thereafter, at the completion of my husband's subspecialty training fellowship, we moved to Florida. Armed with only education, love, and a joint passion for medicine, we embarked upon our journeys of raising a family and developing our professions.

While my path was punctuated by the birthing and raising of three children, I ultimately developed a twenty-plus-year career in diagnostic radiology, including over ten years as a solo practitioner at an extremely busy, extraordinarily popular, and professionally satis-fying mammography and clinical breast imaging practice—a practice that, with the assistance of bank loans, I designed and created myself. I built and nurtured this practice while being married to a physician and raising three children. This was a unique practice.

In addition to the imaging components of breast disease diag-nosis, I offered hands-on clinical assessment and the face-to-face per-sonal attention and emotional support necessary for the total care of women's breast health.

My practice exploded. It became extremely difficult to get an appointment with me, and it became necessary to schedule well in advance. I was very, very busy and very, very happy. I was really help ing people, and I knew it. I was deeply involved in the lives of my patients, and they sought my advice—both medical and personal. People kissed me on the street and thanked me for saving their lives, often in front of my children. As a wife and mother, I became a master of efficiency as I learned how to rank the importance of personal tasks and how to delegate the responsibility for their fulfillment. Other physicians sought my opinions, I was asked to write articles and give lectures, I received multiple community honors, and I was asked to sit on the boards of directors of organizations. The community treated me as though I was a pillar of knowledge. It was both a professional and personal dream come true. And suddenly, it was all over. I was diagnosed with multiple sclerosis.

Multiple sclerosis is a peculiar disease. Since my diagnosis in January 2001, I have often been approached by numerous well-meaning people telling tales of friends with MS (he or she had it really bad) who experienced a miraculous cure. The treatments often involved following a new diet, which was either very restrictive—absolutely no dairy, gluten, refined sugars, etc.—or very lopsided: one must only eat organically grown vegetables (preferably no meat and absolutely no red meat whatsoever!) with a preponderance of beans and leafy vegetables. Some of the meal plans were low-fat, low-glycemic index diets, undeniably sensible for cardiac health although not clearly of direct benefit to the condition we were discussing. Most of the diet stories ended with the protagonists throwing away their canes and running the New York Marathon (or some such thing). One person had a story about an unusual but exhaustive exercise regimen that an actual person with MS designed. The creator swore that it helped him so much that he felt duty-bound to make it available to other sufferers. He, therefore, released an educational CD, which one could easily order online for only $29.95 plus modest shipping and handling charges. Then there were those who had friends with MS, who had left their unaccommodating neurologists and instead visited alternative therapists—often in Canada, Mexico, or Europe—who treated them with such unconventional therapies as injections with various poisons, peroxides, and venoms, or who performed total blood volume chelation (or chemical filtration) to remove all the toxins from their ailing bodies. Often after completing the expensive treatments (if they survived them), these folks would leap from their wheelchairs and dance. I would always thank the storytellers for their advice and would dutifully jot down the names and telephone phone numbers they graciously offered. The reason good friends will tell you these fairy tales is actually comforting; it is because they really do care. Apparently, however, they also know that the medically accepted knowledge about the disease and its treatment is similarly unclear and is decidedly less optimistic.

Multiple sclerosis is a difficult disease to typify as it takes many forms, with significant variability even within each group. No two sufferers have the same condition (although often, the symptoms can overlap enough to allow for useful commiseration). Even the experts break the disease into several categories, often with unclear boundaries and significant overlap. One described form of MS, relapsing-remitting (RRMS), appears to be the most common. RRMS is characterized by acute episodes of a variety of symptoms (tingling, numbness, weakness, spasms, pain in various places, severe urinary or bowel issues, transient paralysis or blindness, inability to walk, inability to use the hands for either manipulation or tactile sensitivity, difficulty with cognition, diminished level of intelligence, difficulty with speaking, feelings of chest and abdominal constriction, and/or inability to breathe, difficulty swallowing with an aspiration of saliva and/or food, and personality changes including inappropriate speech and/or behavior, in a list that is by no means complete. The symptoms could be mild (and therefore difficult to differentiate from a normal annoyance like tingles from sleeping on your arm) or severe (like blindness in one eye or paralysis of a leg) and impossible to ignore. As the name relapsing-remitting implies, with or without treatment, the symptoms spontaneously disappear within a few days, leaving the sufferer often believing that the problem had resolved and was best forgotten. Then there are those for whom the symptoms start, continue, and progressively worsen. These people have what is known as primary-progressive MS (PPMS).

Actually, all MS is felt to be a progressive disease in one way or another. It is believed that even the people who have RRMS will eventually become progressive—a condition known as second-ary-progressive MS. Most of the medications (Disease Modifying Drugs, or DMDs) prescribed for RRMS are designed to slow down progression rather than to actually treat or cure.

It is my understanding that progressive forms of the disease are biologically different from the relapsing-remitting form in their mechanism of neural destruction, and therefore treatment would require a unique approach. Unfortunately, most of the limited treatments available for MS (as well as the research about new therapies) are directed at the more common relapsing-remitting form of the disease. In other words, if you have a progressive disease…well, at least you'll get the best parking spots.

vividly remember the day in October 1979 when I was a young medical intern at New England Medical Center in Boston. During my senior year in medical school, after applying and interviewing, I had ranked the internship and residency programs in order of my preference. They, in turn, ranked the applicants, and as happens every year in March for fourth-year medical students throughout the country, a computerized match is made. The day of reckoning! In the few months remaining in the medical student's fourth year, the level of anxiety is dramatically reduced. Although I doubt that anyone said this, it was rumored that if someone told you to do something that you did not want to do after Match Day, the appropriate(?) response was FYBIGMI—pronounced fabigmee. It was an off-color acronym. It stood for F—— You, Buddy, I Got My Internship!

I was proud to have been matched at this prestigious teaching hospital where the cases (i.e., patients) were often referred to us from local area hospitals and were sicker, more difficult to evaluate and treat, and presumably more medically interesting than the typical patients at the local hospitals. Additional patients were admitted, which at that time was known as the Combat Zone—an area of crime, prostitution, and frequent physical violence, lending a high-intensity/high-stress/think-on-your-feet flavor to the emergency room. These emergency patients tended to be largely from a low socioeconomic group with little or no history of routine preventative care. They were often part of a borderline or criminal element which provided a degree of surprise (often frank dishonesty) in our attempts to extract the accurate medical history necessary to provide optimal care. In fact, they represented a wonderful opportunity to learn medicine.

As neophyte physicians, we had to assess the patients' clinical examination and laboratory findings, frequently with little or no accurate history. We learned to gather important data from nonverbal cues. We talked to them. We observed their physical responses. We looked into their eyes. Some patients admitted through the emergency department were people with rare, complicated diseases who had become acutely ill. These were patients under the regular care of the brilliant, highly specialized, academic physicians who were our medical professors and attending physicians. It was our duty to evaluate, diagnose, and begin treatment, frequently in the middle of the night. Often one had to hit the library (Yes! Open at night; this was before the internet!) or textbook to brush up on the underlying rare illness before even beginning. By morning rounds, the attending physician (the grown-up doctor who had actually slept through the night) expected a succinct story including a dissertation on the underlying disease, a presentation of the history of the acute illness, the clinical and laboratory findings, medical assessment and diagnoses, and a plan for treatment which we had already initiated. Voilà! Well done, Doctor! Not too bad, except for the fact that admissions usually happened between three and six times a night when we were on call, which for us was every third night with no days off except for an occasional Sunday after morning rounds. Many of these patients had an uncanny propensity to arrive at 2:00 a.m., usually just as you had finished your last workup and were heading to bed in the on-call room (a place as well known for sexual trysts as for attempts at sleep; we were, after all, single twenty-somethings). The beeper would go off displaying 5566—the emergency department extension. Even to this day, that dreaded number generates within me a subliminal panic in me. (Fortunately, today, beepers have been largely replaced by ubiquitous cell phones with cheery ring tones, ameliorating one's personal phobia.)

This is how I learned medicine. Despite the physical trauma, I have to say that overall it provided emotional and spiritual growth. I followed patients who were very sick through their entire hospital stays. I laughed with them, cried with them, treated them, gave them the good news, gave them bad news, spoke to their families, cured them and discharged them, transferred them to intensive care, ran their codes (cardiac arrests), called off their *codes* (i.e., stopped treatment and pronounced the time of death), and signed their death certificates. I learned, I laughed, and I cried.

I'm not sure that every intern and resident is capable of this, but I can sleep standing up—really. The textbooks say that this is impossible, that during deep sleep, the muscles relax making an upright posture unachievable. I learned that during morning rounds (between 6:00 and 7:00 a.m.) when we saw the patients on our service with the attending physicians and presented new data, assessment, and plans while another intern was presenting a case I could lean into the corner, rock onto the sides of my clogs, and reach virtual, albeit brief, unconsciousness. I guess I never achieved deep REM sleep (rapid eye movement—a sign of deep, restful sleep, but the subject of another book), but the brief respite was amazingly refreshing. If only I could have washed my greasy hair, it would have been great. For some reason, I was always even more tired than the other medical interns. The more than ninety-hour workweeks were difficult for everyone, yet I seemed to be more affected. I was dating a second-year surgical resident in my spare time for a while who told me that I had to toughen up and that my schedule wasn't nearly as bad as his was (he was on call every second night instead of every third and was often required to assess patients and perform procedures and surgery having had even less sleep than I did). He was right, but I refused to concede. My response was that in addition to the intense physical labor of call, unlike surgical residents, I told him that medical interns had to *think*. That was my own obnoxious *BS*, of course. He laughed and called me a typical flea, which is the derogatory term used by surgeons for medical doctors. I never knew exactly what the surgeons meant by this, but my guess is it suggests that internists annoyingly flit about the surgeons bothering them with academic details while they (the surgeons) actually got things done (i.e., saved the sick and wounded—a noble goal). That was the more tasteful description. The other definition I've heard is that fleas are the last thing to finally leave a dead body. Far less complimentary.

Actually, I think he thought I complained too much. It's true that residency training after medical school graduation was grueling. Apparently, since my days on the front lines, laws have been passed to shorten the work week and lighten the call schedules, with the goal of making life somewhat more livable for young doctors—as well as for the patients depending on their care. It was a very difficult way of life. I didn't know why, but it was definitely even more difficult for me.

G-O-M-E-R, Gomer. I don't know how long this term has been in use, but it is an acronym I learned from the satirical novel *The House of God* by Samuel Shem, a book published in 1978, which is an exposé of life as a medical intern in a major Boston teaching hospital, laden with dramatically dark (although arguably accurate) humor. It actually stands for get out of my emergency room, and presumably refers to any patient who presents to the ER for fraudulent reasons. If used according to its strict definition, the word would be an expression of righteous indignation; nobody has the right to abuse the emergency room inappropriately, resulting in delayed availability of medical services to the truly needy. Well, every profession has its jargon, and my esteemed profession is no exception. The word gomer evolved to have quite a different meaning. It has come to mean a debilitated, usually elderly patient who is disoriented or unresponsive and admitted for treatment of an exacerbation of a chronic, disabling, incurable illness, which, when successfully treated, renders the patient only slightly less disoriented and unresponsive and ready for discharge back to the nursing home. Every physician in training knew what a gomer was. We had all evaluated them in the ER. Each of us had admitted many of them during our years of training and stayed up all night caring for them. We would take them to the floors, talk to their families, write orders, draw blood, insert urinary and gastrointestinal catheters, culture every orifice for evidence of infection, and respond to their respiratory arrest for which airway tubes, a respirator, and intensive care unit transfer was needed. We would then readmit them to the ICU, write more orders, and evaluate their ever-changing, evolving laboratory values, electrocardiograms, and radiographs. When finally able to retreat to the on-call room to attempt to steal an hour of sleep, we would be constantly awakened by innumerable calls from nursing regarding the treatment of their unstable conditions. Although it's not something of which I am proud, one can understand how a young doctor in training would find an element of sarcasm in staying awake all night to save a gomer. It's not as though my fellow interns and I were not committed to helping the suffering. After all, we were doctors. We were very willing to stay up, work diligently, and care for a sick patient for whom treatment would enable a return to a productive life. But an acutely ill patient for whom the most brilliant diagnosis and successful treatment would return him to his usual disoriented, meaningless life should get out of my emergency room.

Dr. Gerald Feinman was a gomer. He was sixty-four years old but looked much older, with pale flaky skin and sparse gray and beige hair. He had been a robust, workaholic obstetrician and gynecologist in a suburb of Boston and had a large, thriving practice for nearly thirty-five years. There were patients in his practice whose babies he delivered and who had themselves been delivered by him as newborns and whose mothers he continued to care for gynecologically. Although he was well-known in the medical community for his superior surgical skills, all the interns and residents thought that they knew more than he did about the science of medicine (if you didn't think we knew everything, you just needed to ask us, and we'd tell you). Although we smugly believed that we were educationally superior, we could not deny the fact that this man's diagnostic skills were remarkable. He was an excellent physician. A careful physical examination, attention to the history of the ailment, and close observation of the patient's nonverbal cues were all he really needed to accurately diagnose and treat. He completed his residency—night call and all—many years before us, and he remained on call for his patients at night and on weekends throughout his career. We knew more about all the new laboratory and radiological tests than he did; many of the modalities had only recently become available, and this knowledge was now considered part of the standard medical curriculum, but he didn't need them at all.

Dr. and Mrs. Feinman had successfully raised a son and two daughters, sent them all to college (and the son to medical school), and saw them establish careers and marry. Actually, Mrs. Feinman pretty much did it all alone because the doctor was still at the office or on call or trying to get a little sleep. His children had great respect for him, but I'm not sure how well they knew him. Mrs. Feinman loved her husband, but as years passed and the children moved out, she was desperate for him to slow down and spend more time, enjoying life with her. Dr. Feinman loved his wife. They purchased a three-bedroom condominium in Pompano Beach, Florida, and he begrudgingly agreed to sell his practice and retire at the age of sixty-five. He and his wife would then move to Florida and enjoy the good life. Mrs. Feinman planned to decorate the two extra bedrooms so that when her children visited with their spouses and the grandchildren, they would all have a comfortable place to stay. Dr. Feinman's heart attack came two weeks and three days before his sixty-fourth birthday. It was a beautiful, sunny, but crisp Saturday morning in October that can be found only in New England. He was leaving a local community hospital after having worked all night. It had looked as though it would be a routine delivery of twins. The mother had an uneventful pregnancy and was admitted to the hospital in relatively early labor *to play it safe* as she was anxious. Even though many of his colleagues were almost routinely performing caesarian sections on multiple birth pregnancies, the doctor planned to deliver the twins vaginally. He felt that although other obstetricians would do a planned surgical delivery for convenience, there was no medical reason to do this and put the mother and babies through the risks of surgery. This was a second pregnancy. The first child was a young daughter who was delivered in this hospital by Dr. Feinman nearly three years earlier. She was eager to become a big sister as she waited at home with Grandma. The labor was uneventful through the evening, and Dr. Feinman retired to an on-call room in the hospital at midnight. At 2:00 a.m., a man's frightened voice could be heard screaming from the labor room, and the nurses rushed in to see the father holding his wife's head and pointing to the sheets. Darkly stained amniotic fluid continued to gush out of the birth canal (from fetal bowel contents, consistent with fetal distress) while the nurses stabilized the patient (and her husband), checked the monitors, and called Dr. Feinman, the anesthesiologist, and the surgical delivery room stat. With a whirlwind blur of medical activity, an emergency caesarean section was performed with the delivery of two male infants. Although the mother's blood pressure had dropped during the induction of anesthesia, she was stabilized with IV fluids and medication and was fine postoperatively. The father received first aid for an abrasion to his head sustained while fainting. Fortunately, his fall was broken as he was caught in the arms of a strong orderly outside the delivery room, resulting in a minor injury. The babies were evaluated by a pediatrician immediately in the delivery room and again upon transfer to the neonatal intensive care unit. The smaller of the two babies looked good by all parameters and was given high neonatal ratings (called Apgar scores), consistent with a healthy infant. The larger boy did not look good. He was the one causing the darkly stained fluid. His limbs were flaccid, and his skin remained bluish in color. The nurses and doctors in the neonatal intensive care unit worked with him at a feverish pace, placing intravenous lines and putting a tube into his trachea or windpipe to attach him to a respirator that would breathe for him artificially. After stabilization of his vital signs (i.e., blood pressure, pulse, and respirations), arrangements were made to transfer him to a major hospital with a higher-level neonatal intensive care unit for sicker infants. His prognosis—or likely medical outcome—was grim. Dr. Feinman was perplexed. He had seen no sign of fetal distress or any obstetrical complication prior to leaving the labor room at midnight. He spoke at length with the neonatologist (an intensive care pediatrician who specializes in diseases of the newborn) who explained that the distress appeared to have been caused by a late but disastrous complication resulting in diminished blood flow to the fetus, which (at that time) was virtually impossible to predict earlier. He assured Dr. Feinman that there was nothing else he could have done and that this was simply a case of bad luck. At forty years of age, the pediatrician was significantly younger than the obstetrician, yet as he faced the sad older man, the softened look on his face and his comforting hand on the old man's shoulder made him seem almost paternal. He looked at the deep wrinkles on Dr. Feinman's brow, the pain in the shape of his lips, and his reddened, watery eyes. Nearly crying himself, the younger man breathed very softly so that no one else could hear, *There but for the grace of God… go I.*

Dr. Feinman was wearing wrinkled faded green scrubs with a large perspiration stain under each armpit as he walked slowly through the hospital exit and headed toward the doctors' parking lot. As tears fell from his eyes, he was gripped both mentally and physically by one thought, *If I had just scheduled a routine Caesarian section a few days ago…* This was the last thing on his mind before the unrelenting crushing pain came boring through his chest and jaw, and his mind began to cloud forever.

They say that Gerald Feinman was fortunate to have had his heart attack just outside the doors of the hospital emergency room. It fell into the category of a witnessed cardiac event for which prompt evaluation and care were available, usually resulting in a higher likelihood of survival. This was a massive myocardial infarction (i.e., a blockbuster of a heart attack with death of a large percentage of the functional tissue of the heart). Because of this, there was a serious decrease in the ability of the heart to pump blood effectively enough to feed the tissues of the body. For weeks, the talk in the doctors' cafeteria was about how lucky Gerry was and how if this had happened fifteen minutes later while the doctor was driving home, the result would almost certainly have been fatal. Even so, his heart was not beating for several minutes. CPR (cardiopulmonary resuscitation) was performed where doctors and nurses initially attempted external artificial breathing by pumping a latex balloon-type device designed to force air into a mask held over the face. This was followed by the more efficient method of artificial breathing, where a tube is placed directly into the trachea for eventual attachment to a ventilator that will breathe for a patient who cannot do so on his own. At the same time, they pounced on his chest, attempting compression of the heart through the skin and bones to achieve some degree of circulation.

The hope was that the artificially induced circulation would allow blood to flow past the lungs so that the oxygen in the lungs could get into the blood and circulate to the body's organs, particularly to the oxygen-dependent brain. And they saved him. That is to say, he had a pulse and blood pressure allowing for transfer into the intensive care unit. They would not know how much brain function he had left (remember the brain's blood and oxygen starvation lasting several minutes) until later. In fact, he had lost all cognitive function and required full-time nursing care.

He had become a GOMER.

didn't realize that I'd be this excited. It was June of 1979, and a typical, overcast, rainy gray day in Worcester, MA. It didn't matter. This was the day for which I had been waiting for years. I was about to graduate from medical school. Sometime during high school, I had decided to become a doctor. I cannot really articulate why I wanted to become one. I knew that as a child, I hated to answer the classic question, "What do you want to be when you grow up?" posed to me by Aunt Rita and Uncle Ned (and to other kids by Aunts Rita and Uncles Ned since the beginning of time). My response was always prompt and courteous, "I want to be either a brain surgeon or a belly dancer." The effect of this statement was always predictable. The questioner would blush and stammer, start to mumble something incoherent, and walk away. I would turn my head so that they could not see my hand over my face, hiding a slightly crooked smile (which would later become my trademark). I was pretty obnoxious. But what adolescent was not? But today was the day knew that I was actually becoming a doctor. My smile was straight and wide.

High school was easy in Brooklyn. I pretty much focused on drama, yearbook, and boys (my major), and still managed to do very well. Over the years, I established a longstanding reputation as an exemplary student, such that teachers felt obligated to give me high grades, deservedly or not (and often, actually…not.) My family of four (my parents, my brother, and I) lived in a two-bedroom, one-bathroom tenement apartment, and I shared a bedroom with my brother (yuck), who was four years my junior. My parents always complained that I monopolized the bathroom doing my makeup, and I used *a lot* of it. This was the late 1960s.

In the fall of my senior year, the opening of school was delayed for months by the infamous 1968 New York City Teachers' Strike. Although we kids acted as though we were concerned, we were more than disingenuous. Nothing could be more wonderful than an extension of our summer vacation!

Then the unspeakable happened. My parents announced that they had purchased a home in Long Island, and we were moving. They had worked and saved and could finally afford a home in the suburbs and a better life for us. Someone less selfish than a teenager would have been able to see the pride in their eyes when they announced that I would have my own bedroom—big deal. The worst thing imaginable was happening. I was starting a new school in October of my senior year, and to this day, I believe that this is the cause of all my neuroses. (Can I sue my parents?) I had to meet new teachers, make new friends, and catch up academically—two months into the school year.

Catch up academically? Unbelievable. For the first time in my life, I could not coast. Not only was I two months behind in every subject, but the coursework was challenging and far more advanced. The other students were bright and highly motivated, and the teachers were intelligent and demanding. And even worse, I no longer had the *golden girl* reputation that I had enjoyed for years in Brooklyn. Now I was expected to prove myself. I had to *actually* do work! No *A* for just showing up. I had to actually learn how to study: calculus, science, history, literature.

I hated this new school, but it was, in fact, the best thing that had ever happened to me. I learned how to study. I found school interesting and exciting. And I especially liked biology.

At sixteen years of age, in October of my senior year, I was scheduled to meet with my new college counselor. This was actually a session called college planning, where we would review my academic record, discuss my strengths and weaknesses, and discuss realistic college choices. I had never seen this counselor who was very new to the school, and when I walked into Stacey Cooper's office, I expected to find an elderly, slender, petite, tight-lipped woman with a gray bun and a shrill voice like all the other guidance counselors I had ever known. Instead, behind the desk was a man in his early thirties. He had longish, chin-length, wavy, dirty-blond hair, large eyes the color of Belgian chocolate, and somewhat large—but chiseled—Greek-god features. (Nose job?) He had a perfect tan, with skin the color of a latte with cream (Beach? Tanning salon?). He was absolutely gorgeous. I'm sure that my mouth was hanging open, and I hope I wasn't drooling as he raised his slender but muscular six feet frame from the chair, flashed a set of nearly perfect white teeth, and while still smiling extended his hand out to me.

"Hi, Barbara. I'm Mr. Cooper. Please take a seat."

We reviewed my record as well as the colleges he thought I should consider. Somewhere in the course of our discussion, I heard him ask in his soft but strong baritone (I think I was in love), "Barbara, I know that you're only sixteen." (Yes, yes! Please! Go on!) "But it's clear to me that you plan to have a career." (Oh well…I can dream, right?) "Have you ever given any thought to what you ultimately want to do?"

I began to awaken from my lustful swoon as I felt the crooked smile start to spread across my face. He was asking me what I wanted to be when I grew up! I sat tall in my chair, twirled a strand of my thick, wild, curly blond mane, and announced succinctly, "I want to be a doctor."

That was it. I said it clearly and with obvious conviction. I heard the words come from my lips, but I was still not sure that I had actually said them. But Mr. Cooper continued to discuss colleges and majors, and from his conversation, I could tell that he had heard me and believed me. Right then, as Mr. Cooper continued smiling and talking, I knew that I had spoken the truth. And Mr. Cooper did not blush or stammer at all.

Mary McBride was a beautiful teenager. She was tall and very slender with small but rounded, firm buttocks. Like her mother, she had the athletic body of a cheerleader with a smiling, effervescent personality to match. Unlike her mother, however, it seemed that nature was confused when designing her, endowing this willowy wisp of a child with a prominent chest bearing full, soft, shapely mounds of womanhood. Her breasts appeared to defy gravity and were accompanied by a pair of firm, perpetually erect nipples that could not be obscured despite the demure cotton Cross-Your-Heart bras, sensible blouses, and loose-knit lambswool sweaters that she wore. Not surprisingly, she was constantly pursued by almost every boy in the school. When they spoke to her, they would try to be clever and amusing while gazing at her hazel eyes and alabaster skin. They talked about everything and nothing as she laughed and tossed back her endless cascade of soft auburn curls. So rapidly that it was barely detectable, the boys' eyes would intermittently drift up and down, briefly leaving her face to spiritually graze in the holy garden between her neck and her navel. It was there where they would dream of suckling at the nub of the forbidden fruit and, while engaged in animated mindless conversation, would hold their books low in front to hide their unavoidable but obvious physiologic response. Mary's father, James, was a strict disciplinarian and a devout Catholic. Although Mary begged to go on dates with the nice young men who asked her out, James McBride adamantly refused permission. Although Mary cried and accused her father of not understanding, he most certainly did; she had obviously never counted the months between her parents' wedding date and the birth of her oldest brother. Thus, Mary went through high school with a busy academic and cheerleading schedule, several girlfriends, and many platonic relationships with boys. She accepted her father's edict and was content, for the only feature of this young woman as intense as her feminine pulchritude was her chaste innocence. She never guessed that for many of the high school boys in Dorchester, Massachusetts, while writhing in their beds late at night, fitfully trying to sleep, mental images of her lovely face and naked body allowed for fantasies of indescribable bliss. She was a sweet, bright, and caring young woman, so it was not surprising to anyone that after high school graduation, Mary chose to go to nursing school in Boston, after which she became a full-time obstetrical nurse at a suburban hospital. It was here that Mary McBride met a young gynecology resident named Gerald Feinman.

Gerald was not cool in high school. His Jewish grandparents had died in Europe during the Russian pogroms of the early twentieth century, and both of his parents were immigrant Americans. His father owned a bakery in Brighton and worked long hours, awakening every day by 3:00 a.m. so that the bread and pastries could be in the oven before dawn and in the bakery case by sunrise. He lived with his parents and two younger sisters in an old, faded brownstone in the very ethnic, largely Jewish community of Brookline, Massachusetts (and not the rich part of Brookline, as often pointed out by his mother's sister). His parents worked very hard, and they pressured their children to do so as well. They wanted their American children to grow up in America, go to American colleges, and have successful American lives. Gerald was fortunate enough to come of age between America's great wars and therefore was not forced to allow military service to determine his career path. He had silently heard his parents' message. Although he never expressed this to them, he promised himself that he would work as hard as necessary to escape his parents' immigrant blue-collar destiny. Although he didn't realize it, it was exactly what they had hoped he would do. Gerald was intense. Although not the most intelligent student in his class (in his generation, the city of Brookline produced many exceptional Jewish first-generation minds), he was clearly one of the most motivated. He played the tuba in the band and was considered one of the band nerds, which did not help his reputation among the pretty, flirtatious, self-impressed spoiled girls of affluence he would occasionally gaze at with longing. He completely buried himself in his books and, by the start of his last year in high school, found that his grades had put him near the top of his class. It was a joyous time in the Feinman household when, on a warm spring afternoon in his senior year, Gerald received a fat envelope from Philadelphia, Pennsylvania. It contained dormitory information as well as various forms necessary to apply for financial aid. Typed on a single page in the front of the package was a letter addressed to Mr. Gerald Feinman from the dean of admissions at a highly respected university.

The letter began, "We are happy to inform you…" Gerald could hardly remember the rest of the letter. Although there was one girl in Gerald's high school physics class named Lucy whom he dated for a few months during eleventh grade, he went out with very few girls during the entire four years. Lucy had whispered to her girlfriends that they almost went all the way, but she would give no details, and so nobody knew exactly what she meant. Suffice it to say that on that June day, when Gerald walked the aisle to the front of the high school auditorium and received his diploma, he was technically still a virgin. By the end of his freshman year in college, the few women he met were very friendly, intelligent, aggressive, and for the most part, sexually experienced. Gerald, on the other hand, was not. He was overwhelmed by the confidence shown by the women and, afraid of being exposed as a greenhorn, focused entirely on his studies and refrained from dating. He continued to play the tuba and joined the band but did not join a fraternity or attend the rowdy after-game band parties where definite social expectations existed. Once again, he drowned in his books, and by his last year found that he had a nearly perfect grade point average, which was unusual…especially for premed chemistry majors.

It was, therefore, not surprising to anyone when during the spring of his senior year in college, several medical school acceptances appeared in his mailbox. What surprised him, though, was his own realization that he was about to fulfill the impossible dream, for among the many envelopes on his desk was a letter of acceptance from a Boston medical school. He was going home to become a doctor. A broad smile appeared on his face whenever he thought about it. According to Gerald, his sisters, his parents, his aunts, uncles, and cousins, his neighborhood, and yes, the entire first generation of Jewish Americans who hailed from Eastern Europe, he had reached *the ultimate American Dream.*

He would be learning the arts and science of medicine in the hallowed halls of a prestigious North American institution, where, as generations of gentiles had before him, he would achieve the most coveted professional degree of his culture. He was going to the promised land. The first two years of medical school passed quickly for Gerald, as it was, in fact, mostly a continuation of his basic sciences education, a study of subjects for which he was well prepared. He particularly liked his introductory course in physical diagnosis, which came at the end of his second year. This was a subject that was completely new and exciting; for unlike the cold necessities of biochemistry, anatomy, physiology, pathology, microbiology, and pharmacology, in this class, he was taught, for the first time, how to examine a patient. The skills inherent in the art of physical diagnosis came easily to him. While others floundered, here is where Gerald began to readily differentiate normal from abnormal heart sounds, assess the *acute* abdomen (often a finding requiring emergency surgery), and use his stethoscope as an extension of his ears, which, along with his eyes and hands, revealed the differences between illness and health, as taught by his physician-professors. This was not part of the standard basic sciences curriculum, and it was here where Gerald first came into contact with patients. Real people with real complaints: both medical and otherwise. Here is where he learned to talk to, and listen to, a patient. But in contrast to the others, this was a skill he cherished, honed, and refined. In fact, it was a skill he mostly taught himself.

The last two years of medical school were spent on hospital rotations. He would work for several weeks at a time learning internal medicine and surgery and their many subspecialties as a student physician on the inpatient teams. He made rounds, punctured blood vessels and spinal canals, placed tubes in every orifice, and *scrubbed in* on surgical procedures. He would sleep in the hospital and shadow resident physicians on night duty and was flattered when one of these tired, bedraggled individuals trusted him to do anything on his own. He rotated through psychiatry, dermatology, and radiology. He enjoyed clinical medicine immensely, but he knew that he had found his calling when he delivered his first baby (with a senior resident at his side) during his tour of duty through obstetrics and gynecology. He would often joke that it was the only specialty where you could use your medical skills to relieve pain and then hand the patient a prize! After he graduated from medical school and began his obstetrics and gynecology residency at a regional community hospital, it was evident to everyone working with him that, to Gerald, this line was not a joke. Gerald's goals were to not only relieve pain, cure illness, and deliver babies. He wanted to help his patients find comfort…and happiness. He was not a scientist. He was a doctor.

Between his second and third years of residency, he was well-known among the labor and delivery nurses. His fame was not due to his looks. He was tall, skinny, and gawky, and although he was not yet thirty, he began to show evidence of male-pattern baldness (i.e., the medical terminology for a receding hairline and an evolving central bull's-eye of skin at the top of the head.) His personality was not the reason either, which, although gentle and pleasing, was not of the sexy, strong, intensely masculine variety demonstrated by his swashbuckling coresidents. Third, unlike one or two of his fellow young doctors, he was not famous for his ability to woo, seduce, and bed several nurses within the same week (unbeknownst to the young ladies…initially). He was famous for being the best. We in the biz know that if you are looking for a great obstetrician with exceptional clinical skills, don't ask your friend Beth or your aunt Ruth. Ask a labor and delivery nurse.

Gerald met Mary McBride during the first week of internship, and like every other young man in the hospital, he was in awe of her looks. As was his nature, when faced with such a strong attraction, he fought his desire and buried himself in his work. He diligently cared for his patients and treated nurses and other medical personnel with utmost respect. He was an excellent physician and a great guy. Mary McBride found him irresistibly attractive. Through the first two years of his residency, he worked hard, slept little, and dated even less. He remained spellbound by Mary. As he worked with her, he realized that in addition to her dazzling looks, she was an excellent nurse and a sweet, caring person. She seemed so overwhelmingly perfect that he considered her to be out of his league and did not even attempt to pursue her. It was a wonder that he didn't notice that she had a special smile for him, was often the only one to laugh at his bland jokes, and that when caring for the same sick patient, made a conscientious effort to provide the level of care needed to spare him from a sleepless night. Halfway through his third year of training, he asked her out. Actually, he accidentally asked her out. He was talking to her about Fenway Park, and somehow, she thought he asked her to a ballgame, and she said yes. So they went to a Red Sox game, and they fell in love. Actually, they finally admitted to each other that they had been in love for quite some time. For many months, they dated. Their relationship was chaste. After an evening out, Gerald would gently kiss Mary good night and at a *very reasonable* hour, take her back to the house where she still lived with her parents. He would never dare attempt to *go further* although he was dying to do so, and, unbeknownst to him, she was dying for him to do so as well. Initially, Mary's parents were vehemently against her dating a man who was not Catholic. However, after many screaming matches finally acquiesced. After all, he was polite, respectful, and…he was a doctor. Gerald's parents were a little more difficult.

She was a *shiksa* (gentile or non-Jewish woman)! His father beat his chest, and his mother wailed something about his grandmother rolling over in her grave. Much to their surprise, Gerald held his ground. He loved Mary, and there was nothing they could do to change that fact. When the couple announced that they were going to get married, Gerald's mother threw Mary a bridal shower. Mary's mother and her two sisters chipped in.

On a Thursday night two months before the wedding, Gerald was on call and in the hospital. He had a particularly busy day with three complicated deliveries, one postpartum (after childbirth) complication, and a late admission of a young woman with advanced ovarian cancer and intestinal obstruction requiring evaluation, treatment, and surgery. He did not get to the on-call room until 3:00 a.m. and was still in emotional pain from dealing with the woman's distraught husband. They had three young children. Mary was working a double shift and was still on duty late into the night. He was just slipping into dreamless unconsciousness when he sensed a presence in the on-call room. He felt a gentle touch on his cheek and breathed the unmistakable scent of her favorite cologne that caused an immediate tension, albeit pleasurable, throughout his body. When he opened one eye, he could see her smile, not a wide grin but a small parting of the lips, and visually locked her luminous gaze with his own. As she slipped between the sheets and removed her clothing, he felt a happiness he never thought possible. It was here where Mary blissfully gave her virginity to the man she loved. And although he was too embarrassed to tell her, on that night—that blessed night—Gerald gave his virginity to Mary as well.

After a week in the coronary care unit, Dr. Feinman was transferred to a step-down unit or a ward in the hospital with cardiac monitors but less intensive nursing care than in the CCU, which meant he was almost ready to be transferred to a regular ward. The tubes were removed from his throat, he was off the respirator, and he was breathing on his own. He was still receiving intravenous medication and wore an oxygen mask, but his vital signs (i.e., pulse, respirations, and blood pressure) were all stable and satisfactory. In a few days, he was transferred to a regular ward, the intravenous tube removed, and he was soon well enough to be discharged with excellent blood chemistries. His only problem was that he had no cognitive or motor function. Apparently, the oxygen deprivation he had suffered during his cardiac arrest caused major brain damage. He would stare into space, and although he would grimace when challenged with painful stimuli (i.e., pinpricks), he would not respond to voices or faces and showed no evidence of awareness.

He was initially discharged to home, but after a few months, Mary and a private nurse could no longer provide the level of care he needed. In addition to the administration of medications, he needed to be fed, turned regularly, and carefully bathed and diapered. He was continually drooling and had trouble with secretions requiring regular suctioning with a tube stuck in his throat and chest physiotherapy to prevent pneumonia. One day, Mary woke up sobbing. She held the husband with whom she shared one life in her arms and, with tears in her own, gazed into his vacant eyes. Their grown children arranged for Gerald's admission to the nursing home. The nursing home was in Boston, and the internist who was in charge of providing emergency care to the residents of the home had his main office nearby on *Beacon Hill*—an old, historic, stately, cobblestoned neighborhood, the essence of aristocratic downtown Boston.

His office was actually a little closer to Massachusetts General Hospital than to New England Medical Center, which was in the heart of the red-light district. MGH, or Man's Greatest Hospital, as it is affectionately called by Harvard medical students, is one of the major teaching hospitals of Harvard Medical School and, as many New Englanders believe, possibly the best hospital in the world. But New England Medical Center—the major teaching hospital of Tufts Medical School—was no slouch either and had a very strong reputation in both clinical and academic medicine. Gerald Feinman's doctor was a Tuft's Medical School graduate, and the attending physicians on the wards at NEMC had been his professors. He said that it was for this reason that he was more comfortable admitting his patients there, although we occasionally wondered if it was actually due to the fact that he found the brilliant Harvard resident physicians at MGH more intimidating. In any case, he remained true to his school, and when Gerald Feinman developed a high fever on a Saturday night, he was sent to the New England Medical Center Emergency Room. My beeper went off at 2:00 a.m., and when I called the 5566 extension and groaned about how busy I was, the ER resident laughed. "Babs, you're up next!"

My name is Barbara, and, like Elizabeth, Barbara is one of those classic female monikers blessed with a myriad of nicknames. Babs, by far, was my least favorite. The ER doctor was well aware of this fact, and as I began to argue that I had more hits (emergency admissions) that night than the other on-call interns, I could hear the almost gleeful snarl in his voice as he delivered his final edict.

"You're next. Get down here. I have a hot [febrile] gomer for you!"

I scribbled the last order in the chart of my previous admission, slipped my clogs back on, and stumbled down the stairs to the ER. As I tripped over my own feet and skinned my elbow, I recalled that

I had argued with that ER resident in front of an attending physician on rounds a few months earlier. This was payback time.

Clogs were standard attire for the intern. I think the surgical interns started the practice as many attending surgeons wore them in the OR (operating room). I suppose the lack of shoe laces, ease of putting on and taking off, and comfort when standing in for long periods had made them popular.

Clogs became part of the unpublished uniform, and along with white coats, scrubs, bloodshot eyes, and unkempt hair, he told the world, "Hey, I'm a young doctor doing my residency. Don't take it personally if I run past you and don't stop to say hello."

There were many different kinds of clogs. Some were very inexpensive. Although they looked fine, they were usually made of vinyl, which made your feet sweat, had poor construction with pinching at the instep and ankle, and had no cushion or arch support.

The good ones (worn by the New England elite and other higher-income people who believed in *ultra-high* quality and *ultra-low* fashion) were made by companies in England and Scandinavia and carried prices that exceeded more than one-half a week's salary. As a relatively poor (and cheap) kid from Brooklyn who had been born into lower-middle income status, I happily purchased the inexpensive clogs. I bought them on an evening after a thirty-six-hour work stretch, which contained one hour and fourteen minutes of sleep (not in row, of course). I had shopped with my friend, a brilliant and unreasonably chipper Ivy-educated woman who was raised with a better understanding of the finer things than was I.

She bought a pair of cheap clogs as well, probably so as not to insult me. She was an intern like me and had the same call schedule as I did. She managed to get about four hours of sleep when on call while my on-call nights were almost always nearly sleepless. My explanation of this phenomenon was that she was just luckier, perhaps had fewer admissions, or was getting patients with less complicated illnesses. I soon noticed that everyone got more sleep than I did. I should have realized that my explanation defied the laws of probability. I told myself that I was probably more compulsive than the others, a more involved physician who paid greater attention to detail. I now realize that I was deceiving myself. I was just more easily fatigued than the others. I was actually more exhausted doing the same amount of work of equal complexity. I became progressively more fatigued and far less efficient.

The clogs were uncomfortable and were, for me, difficult to run in, and running was often necessary in times of emergencies. But hey, they looked great with my scrubs. Cheap sneakers would have been a better, more functional choice, but would have looked far less cool. I reached the emergency room quickly, asked the charge nurse which patient was mine, and visually assessed the pale, elderly, desiccated man in bed three. His eyes were open, but there was no sign of awareness or cognition. As we occasionally remarked—with obvious but unintended crudeness—*the lights were on, but nobody was home.*

A GOMER I sought out the friendly ER resident who sneered at me only once, then embarked upon the task of *signing the patient* over to me. In crisp, efficient medical jargon, he delivered a brief medical history, history of the present illness, physical findings, laboratory tests sent and received or pending, and his overall assessment.

After his erudite dissertation, he turned to me and chuckled, "So you see, Babs, Dr. Feinman here is a long-term nursing home resident with no baseline cognitive function, who now has a fever and unstable vital signs with laboratory evidence of a bacterial infection. It is now *your* job to admit him, stabilize his vitals, examine every square inch and draw and culture every imaginable body fluid for evidence of a source of infection, send additional blood tests, order and review X-rays, and continuously assess the findings and monitor the patient to determine the cause of illness and to initiate therapy. Remember, all bloods have to be drawn by you and hand-carried to the lab at night. *Of course*, you won't forget the lumbar puncture (spinal tap) to exclude meningitis and be certain to send a urine culture. I believe you'll have to catheterize the patient for this (another nasty smile). Oh yes, I forgot. It's late. The family knows that he's here. You'll have to talk to the family in the morning…sooner, of course, if the patient crashes (becomes more unstable). The ER is pretty busy. I'll probably have another hit (patient admission) for you in about an hour and a half."

I checked my watch. It was 2:45 a.m. Gerald Feinman was on my medical service for weeks. His fever had been due to a urinary tract infection caused by a bacterium that was endemic to nursing homes. Because of this, the group of infecting organisms had been regularly exposed to standard antibiotic treatment and had therefore developed resistance to the usual antibiotics. This meant that one needed to find another less common, stronger antibiotic in order to treat the infection successfully. It was thus more difficult to treat. The therapy usually required intravenous therapy, necessitating inpatient hospitalization, and was often plagued by more serious side effects.

He required transfer to intensive care for four days when his infection caused a severe drop in blood pressure that was immediately life-threatening. The episode occurred on a Tuesday night, actually early Wednesday at 2:00 a.m. I was on call and in the emergency room with a new admission when my beeper went off, necessitating my immediate presence upstairs at his bedside. A few other on-call interns and residents joined me, and along with the nursing staff, we stabilized the patient's vital signs and transferred him to ICU (intensive care unit). Over the next twenty-four hours, we ruled out other causes of blood pressure instability. Given the patient's history, an acute cardiac event was a distinct possibility, but a careful evaluation of his physical findings, x-rays, and blood tests excluded this diagnosis, and a review of the bacterial sensitivities and a change in antibiotic therapy resulted in marked improvement and blood pressure stability over the following seventy-two hours.

Fortunately, we were able to avoid putting a tube in his throat to assist ventilation, as in this kind of patient, it would be very difficult to ever stabilize respiration enough to remove it. Unfortunately, talking to the patient offered no diagnostic clues. He was never alert or even conscious. His facial expression never changed, except when the nurse was wiping the drool from his mouth or swabbing his lips. The patient's oldest son was a gynecologist in Chicago. I would review his father's condition and treatment with him daily, and it was a pleasure to be able to converse in doctor speak. He understood his father's condition and did not require emotional coddling. Although I would speak to Mary and their oldest daughter daily, the younger

Dr. Feinman explained everything to his sister and mother in detail, using all the tools necessary for a doctor who is also a brother and a son. Although my medical job was no less challenging, the social responsibilities were considerably lighter.

One week after the Feinman admission, I was running to a cardiac arrest at night when my right foot seemed to miss the floor. I was airborne. I landed in a crumpled heap, my knee throbbing, and despite multiple attempts, I could not stand. I watched as white coats and green scrubs and clogs went flying past me, along with nurses pushing electrocardiography machines and carts loaded down with trays of resuscitative equipment. Most of these young lifesavers ran around me, and one of the male athletic interns (who ran the Boston marathon on a day off) literally jumped over me as I sat helpless on the floor through the entire code. For forty-five minutes, I remained essentially glued to the gray vinyl tile on ward 6 South while tears filled with cheap mascara quietly stained my cheeks.

I missed morning rounds the next day, for which I was in trouble with the ward attending. I had asked another intern to cover my service for a couple of hours while I had my knee examined in the ortho clinic. This was a favor he granted reluctantly and about which he complained incessantly to anyone who would listen. He did not specifically mean to get me in trouble, but he had been on call the previous night as well and was trying to get his work done as soon as possible. Apparently, he had a hot date that night with a speech therapist he had been pursuing for some time and wanted to get out of the hospital as early as possible. I wouldn't have asked him for the favor if I had known. It never dawned on me that anyone could do our job and actually muster enough energy for a satisfying personal life. I sure as hell couldn't.

They let me jump the line in ortho clinic, and I waited only fifteen minutes to be seen.

This made me feel kind of special; I ignored the reality, which was that they didn't want me to waste time before getting back to work. A busy middle-aged nurse virtually pushed me into an exam room and onto a stool with a torn green leatherette seat, after which a bleary-eyed unshaven young man with greasy light brown hair (was that a gray strand I was seeing?) sat on another in front of me. He wore a dingy, creased white coat with a mustard stain on the pocket, over which was fastened a black-and-white pin that read Jeffrey Bowman, MD. It took me a second to recognize the third-year orthopedic resident. I had seen him running through the halls of the hospital the night before, and I quickly realized that his glazed look was due to hours of work with little sleep.

"Hey, Jeff," I mumbled.

I gave him a weak smile and ran my fingers through my knotted, curly, dirty hair. I knew that I probably looked worse than he did, which would have been quite an achievement. He glanced at the chart in front of him and raised his bloodshot eyes about an inch. I am sure that he saw me, but there was definitely no eye contact. He quickly looked down at my chart.

"Hey, Barb. So whatcha do to yourself?"

I began to tell him about my fall in the halls while running to the cardiac arrest, but he was obviously not listening. He was prodding and yanking on my knee as I groaned in pain.

"Subluxed patella," he announced to no one in particular, which kind of meant a dislocated kneecap. "Should get a film to exclude associated fracture" (i.e., broken bone).

Hearing this, I then expected to be directed to the X-ray department. Of course, I did not anticipate being pushed in a wheelchair by an orderly, which is what would be done for a regular human patient. I was ready to hobble to the elevator.

"Ah, forget it," he again said to the same no one in particular.

"We'll give you a removable cylinder cast. If you're not better in six weeks, come back."

He then bolted from the room. The same nurse that put me in the room came in carrying a long bivalved blue plastic cast that could be wrapped around the entire leg and sealed with Velcro strips that were evenly placed along the length of the contraption.

"Here," she said, extending the arm holding the cast in my direction. "You can take this off when you shower or go to bed. Be sure to put gauze over the skin under it. Oh, you know how to do it," and she dropped the cast on the chipped pink mica counter in the corner of the room next to the leaky sink.

She was already partly down the hall before the door to the exam room clicked shut, and I was alone. I felt a little dizzy. Actually, I didn't know how to do it. I was not an orthopedic resident. Damn it. I was exhausted and having peculiar spasms of my leg. Even my arms felt weak. Of course, I had MS but didn't realize it at the time. MS probably contributed to my fall in the first place. For a brief moment, I noted a strange feeling, which I believe was anger. Couldn't they take care of me a little? I took a deep breath and quickly brushed aside my unacceptable selfish emotion. They were all very busy with real patients here, and I could certainly figure out how to use the cylinder cast.

"After all"—I laughed to myself, indulging in the self-impressed but idiotic chauvinism intrinsic to a resident in Internal Medicine— "if an orthopedic surgery resident could learn how to use it, so could I!"

My muscles loosened. I felt that clearly recognizable flush of arousal as an image of Mr. Stacey Cooper, the high school college counselor, passed briefly through my conscious awareness. He said that I was a smart girl, didn't he?

For the next six weeks, I dragged my injured leg and blue cylinder cast behind me while I diligently performed my regular duties. I could not bend the knee while it was fixated by the blue contraption, and my foot was persistently angulated so that my vinyl clog would not remain in place. I remedied the situation by lacing an old torn canvas sneaker to the foot attached to the injured leg. I, therefore, completed my ultimate fashion statement. Not only did I feel awful, but I looked even worse than usual. I am well aware of the fact that my patients were sick, and those who were alert were appropriately overwhelmingly preoccupied with their own conditions. This was very understandable. I believe then that I continued to care for these suffering individuals with the utmost emotional support while offering my best intellectual assessment. I asked them about their symptoms, discussed their diagnoses, explained their prognoses, and gently advised them of their options. I tried to draw my patients and their families close as we made decisions together. The fact that I could not erase a certain thought from my consciousness was painfully embarrassing; I found it difficult to deal with my own medical problems with no external support whatsoever. Absolutely nobody cared about me; I was not a patient. I wasn't even a person. I was a resident.

In medical school, we were taught that the doctors, nurses, and other ancillary medical personnel were all part of a multidisciplinary health-care team—a union of diverse professionals who worked together to achieve optimal patient care, a group for which the whole would be considered more than the sum of its parts. The message driven home here was that no one professional could be considered more important than the others. This concept, although in many ways true, was presented to us in such a way to squash any feelings of authority, or more specifically, airs of superiority in the resident physicians. As residents, we were expected to evaluate the sick and injured while respectfully seeking the expert advice of other professionals whose authority we acknowledged and whose recommendations we readily incorporated into our treatment plans. Of course, as the doctor, or proverbial captain of the ship, if the ultimate plan proved to be unsuccessful, it would be the resident's fault. Ultimate responsibility without ultimate authority. Taxation without representation. After years of brainwashing, this somehow began to make sense. It served to reinforce the lesson that although I was a useful working part of a machine, as a person, I was not important. Anyway, although I was an important member of the multidisciplinary health-care team, no one ever asked about my obvious injury or how I was feeling. I may have been captain of the ship for medical decision-making and accountability, but as a human being, I was the last in line. I was hurting and needy, and nobody noticed or cared. And I was always unbelievably tired. I suspect this made me cross, as well.

Gerald Feinman was finally transferred to a regular ward. He no longer required the highly technological facilities and intense nursing supervision of the ICU. Although still being treated, his infection was under control. While in intensive care, he had developed acute renal (kidney) failure necessitating dialysis (*artificial* filtration of the blood to mimic the purifying role of the kidneys), as well as breathing problems resulting in inadequate oxygenation of his blood. Fortunately, under the diligent supervision of the multidisciplinary health-care team, he had a dramatic improvement in his kidneys and stabilization of his pulmonary (lung) function. Although his physiologic status continued to improve, his neurological condition—which included the function of his entire nervous system and, most importantly, his brain—never improved. He remained minimally responsive and was essentially comatose. This, according to the nursing home records, was his baseline. His brain function had been diligently evaluated or worked up in the past with every advanced technological tool available at the time, and the overwhelming consensus was that we were dealing with an irreversible vegetative state. To us, as frazzled, overworked, underslept resident physicians, this meant one thing. We had achieved the ultimate goal. Gerald Feinman was as well as he would ever be, and our success was that we were not sending him out in a box. He was a medically tuned-up GOMER! It was time to try to discharge him back to the nursing home before he became acutely ill again.

It is true that a hospital is for the diagnosis and treatment of acute illness or acute complications of chronic illness. In all honesty, there was not much more that we could do for this patient in the hospital setting that could not be done in his chronic-care facility. To complicate matters, his medical insurance was in jeopardy of being withdrawn as the nursing staff who worked for the insurance company independently determined that the patient no longer required this level of hospital care. Since reimbursement was involved, the hospital administration was very concerned and became actively involved in his disposition. Ultimately, social service, administration, and the *multidisciplinary health-care team* tried everything in their power to get Gerald Feinman discharged. But for whatever reason, the nursing home refused to take him back. I had two other patients on my service who were disposition problems like Gerald Feinman.

Although no longer acutely ill, like all the patients on my service, they still required daily early morning assessment on rounds with the attending (staff) physician. I had to remain aware of their physical findings and laboratory data, and they still had issues for which nursing would page me on a regular basis, regardless of the time of day or night. In addition, I was caring for three unstable patients in the intensive care unit and a ward full of people who were clearly sick, some of whose cause of illness remained frustratingly obscure. To add insult to injury, new admissions were still assigned to me each day and every third night. My ever-enlarging service was reaching critical mass. My cylinder cast was cumbersome, and my knee was persistently throbbing. I began to wonder if I, in fact, had an associated undiagnosed fracture. My legs would sometimes feel very heavy. And I was tired and having spasms and inexplicable tingling. My vision was somewhat erratic. I had recent trauma to my leg. I was also unbelievably tired. Even sleep could not relieve the indescribable fatigue.

I certainly did not realize that my symptoms, although worsened by my frenetic schedule and injury, were consistent with Multiple Sclerosis. With virtually no time or energy to spend on me, my personal hygiene became rudimentary at best. My hair was frequently unwashed with a mass of tangled, dirty blond curls asymmetrically arranged and matted in the shape of my elusive pillow. I did use deodorant daily, but makeup—which, as a narcissistic native

Brooklyn girl, I had used since I was fifteen to overcome my colorless, pale complexion and blonde, invisible eyelashes—became a time-consuming luxury in which I stopped indulging. I was cranky, exhausted, angry, and sad. A sense of panic that I had lost all my energy and that I wasn't going to make it through my training gripped my fragile psyche. My sinking physical and emotional state made me far less socially attractive to my peers, denying me the attention and compassion that I craved. They were all too busy for me anyway. Time would pass. I would tough it out, and my pain seemed to decrease. The numbness and tingling, however, persisted. Although I could always manufacture an explanation, the symptoms could not be entirely explained by trauma.

On my daily trek to the laboratory, I would pass Gerald Feinman's room. One day, I glanced in and saw one of the nurses rolling him over and washing his back. She was softly speaking to him and handled him so gently that I had to smile. Sheila was a very good nurse. She was not really beautiful but had an interesting, expressive face, which was lightly freckled and framed by short, coal-black hair cut in choppy layers. One would have to admit that she was cute. In her late twenties or early thirties, she was happily married to a moderately successful businessman for about five years. Her petite, slender appearance belied her physical strength, and she rarely called for assistance while attending to her patients. Sheila did not have to work for the money as her husband could easily support her, and according to the nursing station *gossip patrol*, he had asked her to quit on multiple occasions. She refused to stop nursing because she loved it. She was clinically astute and could assess the seriousness of a patient's problem instinctively. When she called me because she was worried about a patient, I knew enough to stop what I was doing and run to her side. I often wondered why she didn't go to medical school. Apparently, she was raised in a culture where women did not become physicians, and she never even considered it. She truly loved caring for people. She would assess orders written by interns—neophyte doctors who knew less medicine than she did. It would not faze her at all. She would gently advise the young resident of her recommendations in a way that did not make the doctor feel inadequate and, in doing so, taught many an intern with her clinical knowledge and nonthreatening demeanor. Although reluctant to do so, her husband agreed to a compromise. By reducing her work hours, she could minimize the time that their three-year-old would spend in day care, and, even more importantly, would still have the time and energy to attend to her husband. I would chuckle whenever I thought about it; Sheila taught me the true meaning of the *multidisciplinary health-care team*. I would bark orders to nurses while monitoring the cardiac rhythm when a patient was clinically *crashing*, and a quick glance at her approving face gave me all the confidence I needed. Surprisingly, I found the fact that Sheila liked me to be important. She took this job seriously, and she treated me well. I guess I couldn't be too bad.

It was a Friday in December, and I was making my afternoon rounds. I had heard from social service earlier in the day that the nursing home was finally willing to take Gerald Feinman back. This was a wonderful day. Through the window in his room, I could see the sky, which was grayish blue as dusk was settling in and as snow flurries began to fall over the dirty streets of downtown Boston. The temperature outside had dropped precipitously, and the sputtering hiss of the radiator in the patient's room could easily be heard as it desperately tried to maintain a comfortable level of warmth. It was much too hot. As I walked into the room, I reached into the pocket of my green scrubs and found a knotted rubber band. I quickly used it to tie up my hair which had a cooling effect on my moist neck.

As I washed my hands, I could hear Sheila cooing, "Dr. Feinman, please excuse me, but I have to roll you over to wash you." She continued the one-way conversation as she laughed. "I'm sorry, Dr. Feinman." She reached around him. "You know that I have to do this so you don't get bedsores." A shy flutter of her eyelids was followed by a slowly evolving grin that exposed white but slightly crooked teeth. "I remember that you are particular about how this is done for your patients. You taught me well!" As I dried my hands, Sheila turned and saw me. I'm not sure, but I think my mouth was agape. She was speaking to this comatose patient as though he was alert and oriented, as well as with a degree of respect usually reserved for those in supervisory positions. She turned to me with a sympathetic expression.

"Hi, Doctor."

As she handed me the patient's chart, I could see the empathy in her eyes as she looked at my disheveled hair and unironed blouse. I quickly thumbed through the laboratory results. Immediately launching into medical lingo, Sheila rapidly fired all the relevant patient data, including vital signs, fluid input and output, physical findings, and laboratory results, after which she advised me of her clinical impression.

"Oh," was my erudite response as she then embarked upon a discussion of his wife, Mary, and her absence. "I'm pretty worried about Mrs. Feinman."

Sheila's eyes looked moist. "She is very depressed. Also, she is not coming by anymore, and I think Dr. Feinman really misses her."

I did not respond. I looked for a sign on her face to suggest that she was joking, but there was none. This was unbelievable. I immediately approached the patient and silently began to examine him. I applied my stethoscope to the front of his chest to listen to his heart sounds. As I carefully assessed the beats and rhythm, my eyes absent-mindedly drifted to his face. The eyes were fixed open and filled with an ointment to keep the membranes from drying out. His face was turned to the left, allowing his bubbling saliva to pool on the pillow as it dripped from his mouth. The lips took the shape of an O as his tongue slightly but asymmetrically protruded downward and out of the corner. A thought jumped into my mind. I tried to erase the insensitive reflection, but I could not help but remember the book *The House of God*, which was written by a doctor with the pseudonym Samuel Shem. In the book, this was known as a *Q-sign*, which was considered to be indicative of an advanced state of *gomerism*.

My eyes squinted shut. Sheila helped me turn the patient so I could listen to his breath sounds. There was a distinctive rattling sound at the lung bases. I shuddered as I confirmed this finding. It was consistent with the abnormal sounds of his heartbeat. Oh no. *This was congestive heart failure.*

As a simple explanation, congestive heart failure, or CHF, is the loss of the heart's ability to adequately pump blood, resulting in diminished flow to organs, including the brain and kidneys. In addition, it causes a backup of blood and fluids, resulting in swelling of the feet and legs and, most problematically, fluid in the chest and lungs, which can make breathing extremely difficult, and renders breathing inefficient for delivering oxygen to the blood. I'd like to say that my dismayed reaction was based upon deep caring and empathy, but it was in fact rooted in selfishness. He could not be discharged with this new development. "What happened, Gerry?" I whined as I yanked his hospital johnny aside to view the swelling of the dependent portions of his body. Sheila was visibly alarmed as she pressed her finger into the swollen skin to reveal a persistent dent. "Pitting edema!" I groaned. This finding again confirmed the diagnosis. "Congestive heart failure! Isn't he on low-salt feedings?"

I was breathing fast. I couldn't get enough air. When I became anxious, I felt as though there was a spasm in the muscles of my chest wall that would not allow for deep inspiration. Without realizing it, I would firmly plant my fist into my upper abdomen directly below my breastbone, a maneuver I had used many times in the past. This would help me breathe. I now think that I was probably assisting my diaphragm to overcome the spasm in my chest muscles, another symptom that was likely caused by my heretofore unknown diagnosis: multiple sclerosis.

As my eyes drifted toward the patient's abdomen, I quickly inspected the well-placed feeding tube that had been surgically implanted into the stomach through the skin. All I could think of was the fact that after all this time and effort, I would not be able to send this chronically comatose patient back to the nursing home.

As I grabbed the chart and began to scribble orders, I continued to mumble, "When did this develop, Sheila?" I felt a rush of adrenaline as my face became very hot. My chest felt tighter, and my right leg felt a little weird. "Gerry, why are you doing this...*to me?*" I felt a hand grip my arm, which was holding my pen. The grip was so firm that I could no longer write. "Look at me." It was a low-pitched, gravelly voice I did not recognize. I turned and saw narrowed catlike eyes and a blanching grimace as anger gripped Sheila's face.

"How dare you speak that way to Dr. Feinman!" Her lower lip was quivering. "How old are you? Twenty-six? Twenty-seven?" She was shouting now. "Dr. Feinman was taking care of people for longer than you have been alive!" Her face began to soften a bit. "He was my mom's obstetrician over thirty years ago. He delivered my sister and me!" She quickly continued, "I was malpositioned when Mom went into labor, and my delivery was very difficult." Her eyes widened. "Without Dr. Feinman and his gentle, expert care, we both could have had serious complications...or even died!"

Sheila's hands were moving to emphasize the words as she spoke, "Mom said that he was wonderful and that she never knew just how much danger we had been in until his nurse accidentally told her months later. You know, Dr. Feinman really understood what it meant to take care of someone." Her chocolate-colored eyes were slowly filling with tears. "Much later, when I was a teenager, he diagnosed mom with ovarian cancer." She was silent for about ten seconds, but it seemed like an hour. "This was an awful illness for Mom. It was awful for all of us, really." She clamped the urinary catheter, disconnected the used drainage bag containing a small amount of dark, amber fluid, and attached a new one. "Over the course of several years, she underwent multiple surgeries performed by Dr. Feinman. Later, she endured the chemotherapy treatments he recommended as she tried to live...and she did live for much longer than anyone expected." She poured the dark urine into a calibrated tray. "Dr. Feinman was at her side, offering his expertise, as well as his kindness, comfort, and understanding...every step of the way." She checked the fluid volume in the tray and carefully recorded the number in the output column on the front of the patient chart. "When we were losing Mom"—she closed her eyes and took a short, wet gasp as she closed the chart—"when we *lost* Mom, he was there for us too."

There were then about thirty very long seconds of silence. We both stared at the floor. The institutional gray-speckled linoleum tiles looked slightly warped, and the grooved pattern did not flow properly. It was obviously a poor installation job. I looked up. Somehow, I managed to find my voice although it had become barely audible, "I didn't know…"

She abruptly held her hand to my face as if she hadn't stopped speaking, and I had interrupted her. "When I became a floor nurse at nineteen, he recognized me!"

She was talking very rapidly now, "And he treated me like a daughter. He taught me about diagnosing, treating and curing ill-ness…as well as how to give gentle palliation when cure"—her eyes glazed over—"was not to be." She continued more slowly, "His patients loved him. He and his patients taught me more clinical medicine than any intern"—she looked me right in the eye as she spoke—"could learn in years."

It was clear to me that Sheila loved this man like a father, or perhaps a beloved teacher, both of which he had been to her.

"And"—I flinched when she continued, rousing me from my reverie—"he was like this to so many people. He gave 100 percent all the time." She was smiling now. "I guess he was quite a guy," I interjected wanly.

She turned toward me abruptly, anger again engulfing her fea-tures as her cheeks flushed crimson.

"Quite a man."

Her nose was now a few inches from mine, and her voice became shrill. I may have been raised in an ethnic section of Brooklyn where physical closeness during casual social interactions was considered appropriate, but nonetheless, she was well within my personal space.

"Quite a doctor." She stepped back a few inches.

"And it's *is,* not *was.* He is a wonderful doctor, a wonderful human being."

My eyes drifted toward the contorted, drooling face on the pillow. She straightened his johnny and adjusted his blanket as she spoke, her eyes now nowhere near mine. "And he's not Gerry to you." She spun around like a military cadet and stood nearly as stiffly, her back slightly arched. She weighed barely ninety-five pounds, but the force of her words nearly knocked me down.

"He is *doctor* to you."

She was scolding me. I felt myself unconsciously cower, as if my mother was reprimanding me for breaking curfew.

"He was delivering babies and taking care of his patients years before you were born. He will always be Dr. Gerald Feinman."

She stood erect while breathing deeply. Her voice muffled, softening to the point that it was barely audible. I thought that she might be crying.

"*And…I will always call him doctor.*"

Her body relaxed.

"Because that's who he is."

She walked toward the glass cabinet on the wall to get a needle, syringe, and the medication I had ordered to reduce the fluid in his lungs. The only sound in the room was the soft squeak of clean white rubber-soled nursing shoes. Suddenly, her voice seemed to recover some of its timbre.

"If you try hard, you might be lucky enough to become half the doctor that he is."

Her head tilted toward me, and as the look of anger was replaced by a smug superciliousness, she puffed, "When you grow up!"

After six weeks, the ortho clinic told me that I no longer needed the cylinder cast. Although physical therapy was usually prescribed in follow-up, because of my hectic schedule, I was given a set of exercises instead and told to rebuild my atrophied thigh muscles by exercise and use. My knee was still hurting, but I was told that this was most likely from disuse and that this should improve with time. My leg was somewhat weaker because of the disuse of the muscles, but after a while, I regained motor strength. The low-grade knee pain, however, never completely resolved although the numbness and tingling improved somewhat. As I was used to discomfort, I simply took Tylenol and ignored the discomfort. I just didn't have the time, and as everyone kept telling me, I was probably just being a crybaby, anyway. As I looked at my skinny, wasted, pale leg (which was covered with amber-blond hair nearly an inch long), I realized that it was definitely time to shave my legs.

After my ortho visit, I rushed to the cardiac floor where I was working that month to relieve the intern who washed been covering for me. This was quite a busy rotation. A patient with a severe, emergent cardiac episode was admitted to the coronary care unit, or CCU, for stabilization, treatment, and disposition. If the patient was doing well, he would be transferred to the cardiac floor where he could still be closely monitored by telemetry (i.e., hooked up to a beeping EKG machine that could be viewed [and heard] in the nursing station by highly trained personnel). The patients on this floor were more stable than those in the CCU, where they had almost one on ongoing care. Those transferred here no longer required such intensive supervision although they were far from stable. These patients had an occasional tendency to develop life-threatening cardiac arrhythmias (severely irregular heartbeats) or to suffer cardiorespiratory arrest (cessation of circulation and breathing), at which time doctors and nurses would rush to the bedside to provide the immediate intervention needed to prevent death.

These events showed no regard for the time of day or night. I smirked as I realized that my leg would be getting exercise and use. I was on call that night. I shook my leg to relieve the tingles in my right foot. It was as if my foot was persistently asleep. I couldn't walk correctly, and my right lower extremity muscles felt as though they were not completely under my control. I assumed that this feeling was related to the injury and the casting, with decreased and pro-longed atypical use of the leg muscles. I now realize that it was not. My right leg was not functioning correctly because of faulty wiring— my undiagnosed neurological condition. Maybe that had something to do with why I fell. But the tingles in my hands only lasted a few days. That night on call was a typical night. I had about four patient admissions from the emergency room. Three of the cases were rela-tively easy to evaluate and manage, but one was complicated, both intellectually and emotionally. She was a forty-six-year-old woman with a husband and three teenage children.

By all reports, she had been healthy until about two weeks prior to her admission to our hospital, at which time she developed severe chest pain resulting in admission to her local hospital, where she was treated by her family physician. They tested her and excluded the possibility of a heart attack, and diagnosed pericarditis, or inflam-mation of the tissues around the heart. Treatment was initiated, and the cause of the pericarditis was still being investigated when she began to deteriorate. Her red blood cell and platelet counts (plate-lets are needed for proper coagulation or clotting of the blood) were dropping, and she had started bruising. Platelets were transfused. Later that evening, it was noted that her kidneys were beginning to fail. The local doctors were perplexed. At eleven o'clock that night, she was transferred to New England Medical Center. At midnight, my beeper went off and displayed the dreaded numbers, 5566—the emergency room. I called the emergency department and asked for the emergency medical resident on call. The nurse told me to wait a minute, that the ER was packed with many acute cases, and the doctors were running ragged. After about five minutes, he picked up.

"Babs."

It was Mean Mike—a good-looking, intelligent junior resident whose medical acumen was only exceeded by the supercilious demeanor he directed toward all interns he considered his intellectual inferior. It was clear to me that, to him, I fell into this lowly category. The image of the stern rebuking I had endured last week, when Mike sneeringly told me what he thought I was doing wrong while he unabashedly stared at my chest, came to mind. At resident meetings, where the house staff (resident physicians) would review challenging cases, I often caught him staring at me. It was obvious that he found me attractive. It was apparent as well, however, that his ego ruled his libido, and as he considered himself far superior to all of us as a scientist and physician, he would never lower himself to my level by seeking my social acceptance. In doing so, he would be risking rejection by me, his intellectual inferior, which, for him, simply did not compute.

It was well known that he was disappointed in his *internship match* at New England Medical Center, and he believed that it was an administrative error. As far as he was concerned, he belonged at Massachusetts General Hospital, which was here in Boston, too, and was among Harvard Medical School's most prestigious teaching hospitals. But much to his chagrin, he matched here. He was now here, with us as equals, a description he would constantly strive to disprove. This anxious young doctor on the phone was not the Mike I knew and disliked so well. He was very different this time. He sounded worried and was not his usual unctuous, obnoxious self.

"Sorry, Barb." (Barb? He never called me a civilized nickname before.) "I need you to come down right away to take this patient to the ICU" (intensive care unit).

He was clearly concerned, uneasy.

"I have a sick one here."

His voice had a gentle, almost collegial intonation like he was requesting my assistance. "Started with pericarditis or inflammation of the tissues around the heart…now an impending multisystem failure."

He took a deep breath.

"Possible causes? Maybe it's viral or underlying *connective tissue disease*, vasculitis—" He started to mumble. Over the telephone, I could hear his rapid breathing and the frantic rustling of papers as I realized he was rummaging through the woman's voluminous outside charts. "Maybe a drug reaction…" He gulped as though he had just thought of this possibility. "What are the meds she is on…? What was she recently started on…?" He was still talking, mostly to himself, when I began to speak.

"Michael, hang up and go back to the patient. The ER is busy. I'll be right down to relieve you. I'm on my way."

When I put down the telephone, I could hear him take a breath and mutter, "Thanks…"

As I ran through the halls, I smiled to myself. I knew that he really meant it. As annoying as he usually was, he was an excellent doctor. I smiled on the inside and thought that he probably should have been accepted by MGH.

As residents, we were overworked, long-suffering young physicians in training, and we often felt very sorry for ourselves. We were tired and often selfish when dealing with each other. I seemed to be the most exhausted of us all, and my constant complaints were often met with irritation.

"Jeez, we're all working hard. What did you expect? Just suck it up!"

We would occasionally indulge in gallows humor, which is the telling of tasteless jokes about illness, which arises out of a need to relieve the stress intrinsic to the profession and the emotional strain of training. But in actual fact, we all truly wanted to save lives and relieve suffering. And with the presentation of this critically ill, relatively young, previously healthy mother of three teenagers, whose diagnosis and treatment were elusive and for whom time was of the essence, we shifted into fifth gear. When it mattered, our personal needs, neuroses, and social maladjustments dissolved. We worked together. We did what had to be done. It was later that same night (or morning, I should say…it was 3:14 a.m.) when a code 99, or cardiopulmonary arrest, was announced overhead and in all the on-call residents' rooms. Although excruciatingly meticulous, as always, I was very sluggish, slow, and fatigued but still conscious, diligently writing up my last patient admission. Nonetheless, whether asleep or awake, busy or relaxing, eating, talking, or using the restroom, beepers went wild. Most of the young doctors on call were already asleep in their on-call room. All the residents and interns in the hospital leaped to our feet and ran to the bedside of the patient in trouble. Thanks to a stroke of technological genius available at the time, the floor and ward where the patient was located were included in our alarm call, continuously flashing on the beeper screen like an ominous warning, suggestive of the blinking numbers on a time bomb. You could see interns and residents running through the halls, leaping up flights of stairs, and tearing around corners, many of whom were still pulling up socks or buttoning clothing as they ran. The only words you could hear them say were "Which room?" or "Which bed?" or "Underlying illness?"

Nurses and resident doctors were running with a tidal wave of white uniforms and green scrubs, like a storming ocean of white caps and churning algae. There was an audible squealing of rubber-soled shoes. There would occasionally be responses to random questions. These would consist of one or two words, all uttered while hauling equipment and IV bags, pushing crash carts loaded with resuscitation equipment and medications while dragging electrocardiogram machines—whose wheels sounded like squawking wild birds over the scratched gray linoleum tile. As I entered the room, I saw a few interns and residents who had been close by and who had arrived on the scene first, whose clothing and hair were disheveled but whose faces appeared alert. They were starting intravenous lines, clipping EKG leads in place, and performing CPR, cardiopulmonary resuscitation, with chest compressions, and artificial ventilation using a mask and compression bulb. The interns and I followed the orders barked by the second-year resident who was watching the EKG rhythm strip, which told him how well (and if) the patient's heart was beating.

The anxiety level was high, but nobody stopped working, and although my legs felt very weak (which I *thought* was because I had recently removed my cast), I had relatively normal feeling in my hands. I sat on the corner of the bed and punched a syringe into an artery in the patient's groin to obtain arterial blood gas. This would determine the oxygen content of his blood—a value that would need to be optimized to save him. Within minutes, the anesthesiology resident pushed to the front of the bed. While a nurse extended the patient's scrawny neck the resident inserted a thick *endotracheal tube* into the patient's breathing pipe through his lips that, although very pale, had now taken on an indigo cast. We could then aerate the lungs…first by squeezing a rubber bulb attached to the thick tube by a coil of clear latex hose and later (if the patient survived) by attaching the endotracheal tube to a mechanical ventilator (or artificial breathing machine). As I threaded an intravascular line into his femoral artery, I glanced at the glazed eyes and open mouth of the old wizened being on the bed who had dried saliva streaked on his left cheek and a small, partially dried collection of mottled spittle directly in front of his ear.

It was Dr. Feinman.

The resuscitation attempt, or code, was terminated after a lengthy but unsuccessful attempt at revival. His cardiac rhythm could not be restored, and an examination of his pupils was consistent with irreversible loss of brain function. These factors (as well as several others) told us that despite our valiant efforts, this patient, Dr. Feinman, had, in fact, *officially* died.

The nurses detached the equipment (i.e., tubes, IV lines, oxygen, EKG leads, urinary catheter) from the deceased patient. The emergency equipment was wheeled away, and the charge nurse was busily completing her notes in the chart. The diligent job of cleaning up had begun. The patient's room, which only fifteen minutes earlier had been throbbing with a crowd of busy young doctors, nurses, and technicians—ah yes…the multidisciplinary health-care team—with many barking orders, others shouting results and findings, and all feverishly attempting to diagnose and treat—was now eerily quiet. Only a few people remained in the room, each of whom continued to push on. They were efficient in their work, but in stark contrast to thirty minutes earlier, they did it silently. Everyone remaining had the glazed, disheveled look of someone coming off amphetamines or speed, and in effect, we were. Our natural adrenaline rush was abating. We were in a dazed state, needing to acknowledge our defeat by death yet not allowing ourselves to be defeated. We would achieve this by continuing to work as we were trained, knowing what we had to do to complete our tasks. Creative diagnostic or therapeutic cognition was no longer possible, and fortunately, it was no longer necessary. We could function as automatons, continuing to perform our duties without exposing our fragile souls. But we continued working. We may have still been in a specialty training program, but nonetheless, we were doctors.

The medical resident who was now in charge of Dr. Feinman's care (he was no longer a patient on my service) was at the nursing station talking on the telephone with Dr. Feinman's son. For some inexplicable reason, I found myself lingering in the patient's room longer than necessary. Dr. Feinman's mouth was opened roundly, and the tip of his tongue asymmetrically protruded just slightly beyond the bluish, swollen lips. Ashamed, I lowered my head and squeezed my eyes shut as I tried to erase the incredibly undignified thought from my mind.

The Q sign.

As I slowly raised my head, my eyes linked with his, which were now fixed in a *blinkless* void. I could feel the lifeless eyes staring deep into my soul. I shuddered to sense a link with this dead man. As I looked down at my scuffed clogs and shifted my feet, I thought about Sheila, the nurse who had told me about the living Dr. Feinman, and I had mixed emotions. Although I know that she understood and agreed with the lifesaving methodology of modern medicine, I was glad that she was not here to see the indignity of this man's final moments as we tore and prodded his flesh in our attempts to beat life back into him. But...I was sorry that she was not here to say goodbye because I knew that she would have done so. Here lay the remains of a man who gave boundlessly to everyone he touched. He loved and cared for his wife and family; everyone who knew him realized this. But his affection for his patients might have gone even deeper. These were people whose lives he held in his hands, and he handled them delicately—with utmost care and consideration. And they trusted him implicitly. He made them feel safe. To these hundreds—no...*thousands* of patients—he would always be the wonderful Dr. Feinman.

My fingers and toes were numb. I shook my right leg in an effort to relieve the pins and needles as random sleep-deprived thoughts kept racing through my brain. There were many days and nights that I felt like I couldn't do it. I couldn't maintain the sense of selfless caring that this man had achieved. It was 4:00 a.m. I was absented-mindedly pulling the knots out of my unwashed, tangled, dark blonde-mousy brown hair and running my tongue over the film on my unbrushed teeth. My breath actually tasted bad. I desperately wanted nine hours of uninterrupted sleep. I wanted to do nothing for two days except sit in front of the TV and watch reruns and eat popcorn and ice cream. I wanted to go out to restaurants and to dance clubs, to get my nails done and my hair professionally highlighted, to leisurely shop in department stores for seasonal, fleeting fashions I had time to read about in magazines. I wanted normal relationships with men, with time to actually act femininely coy and play hard to get rather than quick, efficient *contacts*.

There was far too much human discomfort involved in the quest to achieve the professional and personal goal I was seeking, and I had an uneasy sense of inadequacy. Considering his legend, it didn't seem likely that Gerald Feinman ever had these feelings. As I again looked at his frozen, pale, stiffening body, my eyes drifted up to his lifeless face. I was suddenly gripped by an intense, exhausted alertness like an insomniac urgently scribbling strangely inspired poetry in the middle of the night. I continued to peer into the clouded, open, unmoving eyes. Somehow, the distorted blue lips were smiling at me as the misted, motionless eyes peered deep into my being. I stared at the corpse, and while I felt my mind twist with confusion, my bloodshot eyes burned. Quickly, I wiped a few mascara-laden tears off the side of my face with the back of my hand, leaving a dirty smudge on my cheek. I felt a deep, almost tangible sorrow as I gazed upon the remains of a man who appeared to have sacrificed most of life's pleasures for his career. This motionless cadaver had been a man whose children knew him as the father who was too busy to come to the recital…or to the soccer game. Yet the doctor had succeeded in his marriage. He had been a man whose wife knew him since he was in training and who understood him implicitly. She raised the children to understand that their father loved them boundlessly but that…almost like a clergyman, he had a calling.

Mary's strict Catholic upbringing served her well as she explained the concept of loving sacrifice. Gerald Feinman had been a doctor who was a legend in the community, particularly in the minds of his patients. I looked at his face again. By now, the cyanosis, blueness, had fully encompassed the visage, but his lips were undeniably smiling. My right leg felt weak, so I sat on the bed as I continued to drink in his expression. He had died the first time while facing the sad outcome of an obstetrical medical decision; not the wrong decision prospectively yet retrospectively a very unfortunate one. It was an example of the inexact science of medicine, one filled with a number of undefinable variables. Nonetheless, the doctor's pain for his patients' suffering was very real. This was clear to everyone who had the fortune of knowing him. He had lived through an illustrious and fulfilling career of education, self-sacrifice, and caring. He used his exceptional knowledge and love with boundless generosity…and was equally loved in return. I could feel my body loosen as a sense of calmness began to envelop my being, and the clutching in my chest began to ease. I was breathing more comfortably than I could recall. I smiled as I gazed at the dead body. This man had achieved his goal. Like Gerald Feinman had done years before me, I was learning how to be a doctor. I felt my lips start to shift as a corner of my mouth lifted into a crooked smile. It was going to be all right.

As I was shuffling back to my on-call room, I became aware of a clumping of clogs on the hospital floor. It was a quick but regular rhythm, and the sound was becoming louder as the wearer got closer to me.

"Hey, Barb…"

It was a soft Northeastern city accent. I was unfamiliar with the cadence. It was definitely not a New England accent. I had lived in Massachusetts during the years following college and those flanking my medical school and residency careers, becoming very familiar with the local intonation and expressions. I resided in the towns around Boston before medical school, moving to Worcester (which we so sweetly called the armpit of the state) for medical school at the University of Massachusetts and back to downtown Boston for postgraduate training. I was very familiar with the widened *a*'s and truncated *r*'s of Dorchester and Revere with which the working-class patients in my free outpatient clinics (for free, you did not get a board-certified senior physician; you instead were cared for by a resident in training like me) liberally peppered their speech. It certainly wasn't a New York accent. I smiled sardonically about the dreaded accent with which I was intimately familiar—the childhood accent that I tried to disguise in my own speech for years, albeit in vain. Philadelphia. It was a Philly accent.

I turned to face a very tall, lanky young man with dirty blond hair and patchy stubble on his face. He was dressed like me, in disheveled scrubs, and although mine were fashionably bunched at the ankles, his were definitely an inch or so too short. So much for one size fits all. I recognized him as an intern who was not in my group. He was a trainee at the Boston Veteran's Administration Hospital, the VA as it was known to most people. The VA interns spent a month training at New England Medical Center to experience our cardiology ward and care for cardiac patients under the expert tutelage of our physician-professors. These young doctors brought out an unattractive—actually obnoxious—air of superiority in those of us who were residents and interns at NEMC itself, as we perceived our hospital—Tufts University School of Medicine's major teaching hospital—to be far superior to the VA and (undoubtedly) more selective in the match process. His eyes were huge. They were a shade of blue I had never before seen—a shade of blue much deeper than those I saw staring back at me from the mirror each morning. *Contacts?* I wondered. His lids were drooping, and he was clearly fatigued, but his blue eyes sparkled. He was talking softly, but I could not focus on his words. Instead, I was looking at a smiling mouth and the motion of the lips. He was continuously grinning, and as he spoke, I couldn't help but notice that one corner of his mouth was lifted in a crooked smile!

As I returned the facial expression, I caught several words and realized that he was asking me out for the following night. Laughing inwardly, I realized that, like the rest of us, he was not going to allow a sleepless on-call night, followed by a day at work interfere with the opportunity for social life on a night off. This is how we all lived. As twentysomethings, interns and residents quickly learned that the opportunity for sexual pursuit was far more important than sleeping or eating. I wasn't sure I could handle it that night. I was so fatigued, apparently more than my cohorts, and after a night like this, recovery was very difficult for me. This thought quickly dissipated as I craned my neck to better see the smiling face that loomed nearly a foot over my head. He was cute…and very sweet. I was still gazing into his eyes as I heard myself say, "Sure…how about Chinatown?" and murmured my address and telephone number.

He turned and took two long strides to the nursing station, grabbed a pen from a white cup that advertised antidepressant medication in red block letters (obviously a pharmaceutical company freebie), tore a yellow sticky note off a pad in the corner of the desk, and leaned on the gray Formica to jot down what I had told him. He waved see ya later and was starting to leave as I pleasantly noted that on his ankles, which were clearly visible beneath the short grayish green scrub pant legs, were a well-matched pair of chocolate brown socks, which, although somewhat too short, looked kind of nice. He was wearing clogs. I squinted my eyes to better see his shoes as he started to walk away. They were leather—a tan luggage color. As the small logo on the side of one shoe came into view, I could not suppress a chuckle. There was no question that they were the good kind, the expensive Scandinavian ones.

We went to a terrible Chinese restaurant that he apparently liked; he was a Cantonese fan, and I preferred Mandarin or Szechuan. We ate soggy sweet-and-sour chicken in a viscous translucent pinkish-red sauce with overcooked green peppers, which was apparently his favorite dish. I have a tendency to wolf down my food as I'm always in a rush although I've been told that it is not lady-like to eat so fast. I've often tried to slow down, usually without success. But the plus side to the lousy cuisine was that I had no trouble eating lightly, if at all. As I pushed the food around on my plate while we chatted, I could smile and listen and act like the lady I wished I really was. And he talked and smiled and acted like this was normal. I guess most women eat lightly on a first date! Terry was from South Jersey, which is, in essence, suburban Philadelphia. (Years later, my eldest son described New Jersey as the backup state—a state without its own personality, where North Jersey is culturally and financially suburban New York and South Jersey is merely an extension of Philly.

Of course, this is not *really* the case. Although our son was joking when he made this statement in an attempt to tease his father, he, in fact, raised an arguable point!) Terry told me that he was going into Radiology; apparently, he had been accepted into his residency during his senior year in medical school, at about the same time that I matched in medicine at New England Medical Center. His radiology residency required a year of Internal Medicine internship first, and he was scheduled to begin the residency the following July. He had gone to medical school in Philadelphia—apparently at the behest of his recently widowed mother—and was now excited to have moved to Boston, arguably the *mecca of medicine*. He was doing his internship at the Boston VA. My mind drifted as he spoke. I felt the familiar chauvinistic flush in my chest as I thought about the superiority of my internship. The VA was no match for NEMCH. I tried not to let the smugness show on my face. He didn't seem to notice, thank goodness, as he continued to talk. I was such a bitch. I looked at him. His face was animated, smiling, and boyishly handsome. In the course of the conversation, I asked him where he was going to do his Radiology residency. I knew that Radiology residencies were quite competitive, and it was difficult to get any residency. This lucky VA intern...was he staying at the VA for his residency? I heard it was pretty good. Was he lucky enough to be coming to a Boston area university hospital? I smiled...or was he going to one of the many area community hospitals? I was hardly listening as he responded, explaining how he was lucky to get an apartment on Newbury Street so he could walk to work. Wait a minute...the VA was nowhere near Newbury Street. Terry was cheerfully talking for five minutes about the amazing phone call he got from the Radiology residency program director about how his medical school roommate had answered the telephone, covered the mouthpiece, and started screaming uncontrollably until Terry took the phone...about how he explained to his recently widowed mother that he absolutely had to leave Philadelphia. I was hardly listening as I looked at his animated face. He had obviously shaven. There was a fresh pinkish shaving cut on his left chin although he didn't shave too well with at least one small blondish patch of stubble remaining. His hair was a mess. I was still thinking about his face when I realized what words he was saying, Massachusetts General Hospital. MGH, the crown jewel, was where he was going to be a Radiology resident! Mass General! Oh my god! My self-centered, New England Medical Center, stuck-up balloon was quickly leaking air.

My residency group often talked about residents at the General metaphorically, being cartoonlike angels of medical perfection who could not be real. I suddenly realized that I was probably talking to a medical school genius, one of the chosen few. I was starting to feel embarrassed by my earlier assumptions and considered apologizing, although obviously, I never told him my assumptions. I looked at him and realized that an apology would not be necessary. Terry obviously knew the effect that this information inevitably had on medical people, and he learned to take it in stride. There was no boastful swagger evident as his gentle, smiling, poorly shaven face came into full focus. But those eyes, they were the largest bluest eyes I had ever seen on a man. And they were gazing directly into mine. I looked closely at them; they were intriguing. They would intermittently sparkle and squint into a smile, and they had a distinct, although subtle, look of confidence.

A few weeks later, I heard that Mary Feinman had died. She was walking home from church in the rain one Saturday evening and apparently slipped on the pavement and struck her head. It was dusk, and few people were on the street. Most were either having dinner or getting ready for a night out. She went to pray and to hear a sermon about the heavenly rewards awaiting those who lead a good life. She usually went to church on Sunday morning, and attending the Saturday evening service was not the norm for her; nobody knew that she had gone. Although her children called her several times a week, she lived alone, and nobody was expecting her return. It was uncertain as to how long she had been lying on the sidewalk before she was found by two college students jogging in the rain. Because she was taking blood thinners for a cardiac ailment, she developed a large, rapid bleed in her head, and by the time she reached the emergency room, she was already dead. Linda, the head nurse in the ER, had known Mary for years; she had worked for Dr. Feinman in the past and had attended many Feinman summer barbecues, having enjoyed Mary's cooking and effervescence.

She was crying when the resident on call pronounced the time of death although she insisted that, even in death, during this final hospital visit, Mrs. Feinman had a smile on her face. Everyone knew that this was in Linda's imagination and, in her sadness, her way of dealing with the loss. Dr. and Mrs. Feinman had purchased a retirement villa in Pompano Beach, Florida, about eight years earlier. They bought a three-bedroom, three-bath unit with a huge eat-in kitchen. There were built-in white-painted wooden cabinets and pantries for abundant storage of food, dishes, pots, pans, and numerous cook-ing tools and utensils—none of which were electric. Mary strongly believed that homemade was synonymous with made by hand. This villa was far more than the two of them needed, but Mary had insisted upon the extra space so that the children and grandchildren would be comfortable and often visit, eager to enjoy the Florida sunshine and lifestyle, as well as Mary's cooking and pampering. Although they had not yet moved there as the doctor had not yet retired, prior to her husband's sudden illness, Mary had begun to furnish the villa. Unfortunately, after Dr. Feinman's heart attack, nobody talked—or even thought about—the retirement condo.

It had remained empty, with only the dining room and guest rooms partially furnished. After Mary's death, their children inher-ited the condo. None of the Feinman children wanted it, for even if they were interested in a place in Florida, this condo was in a neighborhood specifically geared toward senior citizens. Given the fact that they were families with children, it was of no use to them. And although they never told their mother this, as it would probably upset her, they didn't even like it. The oldest son, who was a doctor in Chicago, was assigned the task of selling the unit. According to the real estate agents, it was a *tough sell*; a three-bedroom unit was not popular among retirees at that time. These were older folks on a fixed income who were willing to pay more for a two-bedroom than a one-bedroom unit so as to have a spare room for an office or for visiting grandkids but who were unwilling to pay more for a larger three-bedroom unit, which also demanded higher operating costs (i.e., electricity, gas, etc.). In addition, since Mary and Gerald pur-chased their villa, many newer neighborhoods had arisen, and, unlike in New England, where an older home is cherished for its charm and history, in Florida, it is no better than three-day-old bread, ready to be discarded and replaced by a fresh loaf. The new bread may have been baked with highly refined, processed flour rather than with the whole grain, enriched goodness of the older loaf. Yet in Florida—the land of Ponce de Leon and the fountain of youth, the perfect tan, six-pack abs, and tight, surgically enhanced breasts and derrieres—the latest and greatest was considered the best, and newer neighborhoods quickly replaced the older ones in desirability. The more financially secure retirees would regularly sell their old condos and move to newer places to be where *the action* was. In fact, for retirees to settle and stay in the same neighborhood was a sign of surrender, a confession that they understood that they were now on the inevitable road to eternity. Instead of pursuing a newer, more vibrant neighborhood, the next step would be assisted living...or worse.

The Feinmans had purchased their villa well before they planned to move, and it was in an older development. A condominium that had once represented the culmination of Mary and Gerald's dream for the future—a future that could, while surrounded by children and grandchildren, be filled with activities, pleasurable delights, joy, and relaxation—had now become an albatross around their children's necks. Even with nobody living there, the property incurred basic utility costs, condo fees, insurance, and property taxes. To make matters worse, their son, the gynecologist (who had been assigned by his siblings the task of the *condo problem* because he, as his sisters said, had the most business acumen), was in the middle of a messy divorce, and he resented his sisters for not helping with the sale. He knew that his siblings meant well, but dealing with this issue was a big nuisance and interfered with his life, taking far more of his attention than it was worth. He had a crumbling marriage, three teenage children, and a busy practice. He felt somewhat guilty, knowing how much the retirement home had meant to his mother, but he brushed that feeling aside. Although it was probably once a good idea, the villa could no longer serve its intended purpose, had outgrown its usefulness, and had become a burden. After eighteen months on the market, he sold the condo at a substantial loss.

was a second-year Internal Medicine resident physician when the *meltdown* came. I was on call in the hospital and sitting at a desk in the nursing station of *6 South*. I was now one of the senior house staff on call and sleeping in the hospital that night and had first-year interns under my supervision. At night, I would see the patients assigned to my service after the interns. The intern would have also evaluated the patient. They would have written the admission summary and write the doctor's orders in the chart, which would be followed by the nurses. It was my role to provide a more experienced assessment, provide my own assessment and plan, and of course, carry more of the patient-care responsibility. It was my evaluation that was the last word. It was 2:00 a.m., and I was still writing up my 11:00 p.m. admission. I had briefly seen my 1:00 a.m. admission (my fourth of the night), checked the write-up and orders written by the intern, and assured myself that the patient was stable enough to await my professorial exam. I stared at the page upon which I was writing, and although no one else was around, I felt a heavy spur-laden boot crush the back of my head.

The words in front of me were coming in and out of focus, and as I wiped the tears from my eyes, I couldn't seem to completely clear the view on the right. Although I was unaware of this at that time, I now realize that this symptom represented inflammation of my optic nerve, which affects vision. In fact, I was lucky that it did not lead to blindness in my right eye. In addition, the exhaustion was indescribable. I could hardly hold the pen in my right hand, and my handwriting, which I would often joke was so neat and beautiful that you had to check my files to be sure that I was, in fact, a doctor, was barely legible, even to me. In retrospect, I was clearly having an *MS flare* or exacerbation. I lay my head down on the desk for what felt like a few minutes and was jolted to consciousness by a loud, rasping cough that intermittently punctuated the persistent timelessness. It seemed to come from nowhere—a disembodied sound, an auditory hallucination. Except for me, the nursing station was deserted. I looked at the clock on the wall. It was angled slightly to the left as it always was, revealing a discolored, coffee-brown spot on the gray wall, which—if the clock was hung straight—would have been tastefully hidden. My mind was empty except for this awareness: the image of the tilted timepiece told me that I was on 6 South, as the clock on 6 North leaned to the right. The clock's dull, electrical hum was filling my left ear as the ward was otherwise silent save for the occasional punctuation of the air by the bronchial hacking of the chronic lung disease patient in room 637, bed B. My right ear was completely enveloped by the pounding of my pulse. It was 4:00 a.m.

I can't go on like this was the only thought filling my brain. My head was swirling. I continued to hear the whirring of the clock and the barking and gurgling of the incessant cough. *I can't do this.* The thought that I was going to fail knifed through my brain, that I was never going to achieve the goal to which I had devoted most of my life. This had been a goal for which I had struggled and worked and given up personal pleasures and restful indulgences. The thought was one of the most painful of my life.

I was not going to make it.

My hands were tingling, and my feet were numb. I was a failure. I should never have done this. The tears were flowing freely now, and I was choking and gasping with sadness, but there was nobody around to hear or see me. My head was exploding with painful memories of college premed; of organic chemistry, genetics, and histology; of medical school; of the hundred-plus hour work weeks; of the erratic schedule, crummy diet, lousy haircuts, and old wardrobe of an overworked intern; of the parties and vacations I had missed; of the high school friends who had become teachers after college and who now had husbands and babies, of the crummy, superficial, noncommittal sexual relationships; of the relatives who told me that I should not go to medical school and who may have been right. I thought about the day I received my letter of acceptance to the University of Massachusetts Medical School, and while celebrating with my college boyfriend, hearing him ask me not to go to medical school and to marry him instead. I thought that he would never ask, and I was surprised to hear myself turn him down in order to pursue a goal I never really believed I would be offered. And now I was failing. I was in my late twenties, and the realization that I probably made all the wrong decisions was gripping my abdomen, and the pain of admitting defeat to my parents, to my family, to the world was excruciating. Somewhere in the depths of my semiconsciousness, I could visualize ending my life as a solution, as a way to eliminate the agony. I shook this thought away as quickly as it emerged, but I had thought it and could never *un-think* it.

I looked at the chart again, but this time in a dissociated way, as though I was floating above and looking down at the gargantuan patient chart, which I was expected to commit to memory in my diagnostic data bank. It was laden with an endless accounting of a man's childhood experiences, medical and surgical conditions, foibles, emotional issues, social inclinations, medications, addictions and preferences, physical findings, as well as X-ray and laboratory data, all in meticulous detail and perpetually evolving. My vision seemed blurry. I was once again experiencing the deep fatigue that I often tried to explain but couldn't—a sensation I have since learned is common in multiple sclerosis, an overwhelming weariness that no amount of sleep would relieve. I had no idea how long I sat there thinking…or not thinking. As I blankly stared at the overstuffed blue folder in front of me, I struggled to regain focus.

There were innumerable discharge summaries describing the patient's multiple hospitalizations for both medical and surgical conditions, each of which attempted to direct attention toward the facts related to the current illness although the extensive mosaic patterns of his numerous medical conditions were inextricably interlaced at all times. I had always believed that to be the perfect doctor of internal medicine, one must fully understand and treat the total patient.

The doctor must consider all facets of the patient, both old and new, to best evaluate the current, presenting illness. Achieving this would be highly commendable and would satisfy the perfectionist nature and educational goals of someone like me, someone with an *obsessive-compulsive* nature, someone who would make an exemplary medical student but who might be an ineffectual practitioner of Internal Medicine. To be a functional internist, one who could function in an expedient manner, a doctor must be able to tunnel his vision toward the problem at hand, directing attention to the evaluation and treatment of same, assessing the extraneous medical conditions only to the degree in which they affected the evaluation and treatment of the problem at hand. I could not do this. While evaluating the myriad of clinical details, I would be overwhelmed by a strange, devastating fatigue, which left me in a nonfunctional haze. I had been a good medical student, having an encyclopedic knowledge of clinical and scientific medicine as well as strong skills in physical diagnosis and laboratory data interpretation. In fact, I was even nurturing and caring with a good bedside manner. But now, while on call in a busy hospital, I could not find the time to efficiently complete the workup of single patient admission, not to mention multiple patient admissions with time left over to get some sleep. I remained caught up in the infinite details of the totality of the patient's condition until I drifted into an exhausted, endless spiral. I was just not effective. And I was just so damned tired—all the time.

Although I was an intelligent doctor, after trudging through the thick sludge of a patient evaluation, I became physically and mentally drained, with a distinct inability to *cut to the chase* to sprint the final few meters. To avoid the acute psychomotor malfunction, my inevitable physiological and emotional crash, I had to find a way to constructively reroute my natural inclinations so that assessment, evaluation, and treatment of a medical problem could be completed prior to my shifting into overdrive. I needed to redirect my exhaustive attention to detail to one problem at a time. The answer had become clear. As this sad realization floated to my consciousness, my entire being began to sink to a depth of fatigue I had hitherto not experienced—a realization that I no longer knew myself and was not sure I liked what I did know.

Today, I realize that I was experiencing the hopelessness of depression although because of this, at the time my insight was limited. For years, I had hoped and dreamed of becoming a doctor. And in my subconscious mind, as well as in the conscious minds of my family and friends, a doctor meant an internist—a *regular* doctor— the one you would call when you were sick. What was clear to me then was one sad, irrefutable conclusion. I could not, and should not, become an internist.

During my medical school psychiatry rotation, I was taught to pay very close attention to a suicidal patient who suddenly appeared happy. They said that a depressed person with suicidal ideation could demonstrate an incongruously peaceful emotional appearance, or *affect*, once he or she had finally decided to act on his self-destructive impulses, once a distinct method of suicide and plan of implementation had been determined. The map of the road toward the resolution of the painful condition had finally been carefully sketched and was ready to be followed. In essence, a suicidal patient with a depressed affect who suddenly appeared inexplicably content should raise a red flag. After my epiphany, I became like such a patient. To relieve the psychic and physical pain of my life, my dream of becoming an internist had to die. And I knew how and when I would kill the dream.

Over the next few weeks, everyone commented how much happier I seemed. Fortunately, this was not due to my having reached the anticipated tragic conclusion. During this time, my relationship with Terry had evolved, and my decision, although life-altering, took a very different path.

After our first few dates, my relationship with Terry blossomed. He had finished his rotation at New England Medical Center, where I was an Internal Medicine resident, had returned to the Boston VA Hospital to complete his internship, and started his Radiology residency at Massachusetts General Hospital. I had heard through the grapevine that he had been something of a womanizer during his internship, and he was uncomfortable dating someone who worked in the same hospital as he did. I suppose he had already experienced the social fallout of breaking up while still working at the same hospital as a nurse or other coworker and decided that it was not worth the risk. In any case, now that he was safely ensconced as a Radiology resident at the General, as a second-year medical resident at New England Medical Center Hospital, I was now fair game. The hospitals are only 1.97 miles apart, but for Terry, these were a critical two miles.

Terry lived in a cramped efficiency unit in Back Bay masquerading as a one-bedroom apartment in the real estate brochures. It was a fragment of a distinguished old brownstone that had been scooped up by an investor during a real estate upheaval and who quickly converted this stately historical structure (that had once been a single home for generations of Boston Brahmans) into multiple minuscule living units (loosely called one-bedroom apartments). A working fireplace would be maintained for old-world *charm*, with additional walls dividing larger spaces into two tiny rooms. A diminutive bathroom was provided. This included a stall shower, toilet, and miniature sink and was good for your diet, as there was no way you could fit into the room if you were overweight. Furthermore, the lavatory could only be reached through the bedroom. I believe this was considered to be a positive feature for single men, as it required a guest to walk into the bedroom to use the facilities.

There was a strip of small dormitory-style appliances applied to a wall of the living room, which was generously (though imprecisely) called a kitchen. The most innovative aspect of this apartment was the bedroom. It was small. (Now, when I say small, I don't mean *smallish*. I mean *very small*.) Let's just say that Terry had a queen-size bed, not unreasonable for a man who stands six feet two. This bed was pushed into a corner of the room and directly abutted a window on one side, a wall at the head of the bed, and the threshold of the entrance door at the foot of the bed. Fortunately, the bedroom door opened (atypically) outward toward the living room and not inward as is typical for bedroom doors. I believe that this construction tradition is based upon modesty...if someone enters the room with the door opening inward, it allows the person in the room a few extra seconds to cover up. In this case, the door opened outward for a very practical reason. If the door was hinged to swing into the bedroom, the bed would not allow for the door to open at all.

The side of the bed opposite the window was approximately six inches from the adjacent wall, which was good because it allowed one to stand with his feet sideways, one in front of the other, and twist the body to open the sliding door of the room closet. A tall person (lucky Terry, unlucky me) could actually reach over to retrieve items of clothing or shoes (all of which of necessity were few in number to fit in) from the mini-alcove called a closet. Along this same wall was the door to the lavatory. As I explained, this room contained the only toilet in the place. It was, therefore, necessary for *anyone* needing to use the toilet to step on the bed to enter the bathroom.

This was initially a problem, particularly in the winter when everyone's shoes were covered with dirty gray slush; however, this was successfully remedied when Terry established a *no-shoes-in-the-apartment* strategy. The window in the bedroom was fitted with the original kind of glass that diffracted light in such a way as to make everything look wavy, suggesting that it was the original hand-blown glass. This feature contributed to *old-world* charm.

Outside the window was a re-painted black wrought-iron fire escape, complete with a twisted, winding ladder extending to just above street level. The fire escape successfully served two purposes: one, it allowed the resident safe egress to the street from a burning building in case of fire, and two, it allowed easy ingress for a burglar who knew which nights the young doctor was *on call* and would not be returning home until the next day.

Fortunately, there were no fires. Only the second of these two functions was utilized during Terry's tenure. But the apartment was on Newbury Street, probably giving it the coolest address in the Back Bay and possibly in all of Boston. It was a wide tree-lined street, replete with sidewalk cafés and elegant restaurants, funky stores, and haute couture designer boutiques. All the best salons and spas graced its streets, and everybody who was anybody in Boston could be seen strolling its promenade any weekday evening or weekend day. And there was nothing more comforting, relaxing, or romantic than, after a harrowing day at the hospital, to lie together on a fuzzy living room rug in the dark, with only the soothing, sputtering, popping light from the fireplace illuminating your lover's face. Terry loved his little apartment. And so did I.

Time inexorably passed, and it became time to renew Terry's lease. He and I had been an exclusive *item* for more than six months when I first broached the question. Although he clearly had the more desirable address, living on Newberry Street represented the height of fashion, social savvy, and *yuppie-dom*. I lived in a rather large modern one-bedroom apartment in a building that stood almost exactly equidistant from our two hospitals. My apartment was significantly closer to Mass General than Terry's place. Although not as quaint as Terry's, my apartment was significantly larger with expansive rooms and closets and a bathtub as well as a shower. A distinctive feature of my place was the beautiful kitchen, boasting a large, high-end refrigerator/freezer and, even more dramatic, a gas oven and stove top with eight burners in a proper array for cooking, which could be the envy of every amateur chef in the downtown area. Although I was not much of a cook myself, I had heard it said that the way to a man's heart was through his stomach.

I chose my words carefully, closely observing Terry's face and body for expressions belying his reactions—both conscious and subconscious. My apartment was clearly a better choice for his day-to-day life; its location would make his pedestrian commute much easier, particularly in the cold, damp, slushy New England winters, which were particularly unpleasant when trudged at night after a long day and evening in the hospital. Its size was a significant advantage. The size of the bedroom and closet allowed two people the luxury of both standing in the room at the same time without even disturbing the bedspread, not to mention allowing the closet door to be open or closed at their whim, making it more conducive to civilized life. And given the fact that we spent most nights together—and I already lived there—the choice seemed obvious to me. In the middle of an unrelated conversation, such that it would be received like a subliminal thought, I subtly questioned if he had considered moving in with me. I observed as his back gently arched while his hands began to clench and unfurl, almost rhythmically. His mouth was closed, and his lips were drawn tight and slightly angled across the bottom of his face like a horizontal apostrophe. One did not need to study psychology to see and feel the tension emanating from him. I knew that if I wanted to convince him to move in—heck, if I wanted to prevent him from bolting out the door—I needed a very persuasive approach. I could feel my crooked smile trying to erupt as I attempted to maintain an appearance of quiet sincerity. I managed to force my devious smile back, knowing the slyness it suggested, as I attempted an ingenuous affect. I *knew* what I had to do.

Oh yeah, I was going to break out the big guns.

"I don't have a car," I began matter-of-factly. "And my building has an attached, enclosed indoor garage complex."

I perfected the timbre and tone of a nonchalant chat with a style of thinking out loud.

"I get an assigned garage parking space included with my rent."

I paused deliberately, carefully observing as his hands unfolded and his head slightly tilted toward me.

Then as if I had just had an epiphany, I continued, "Hey...you have a car. Maybe we could use the space for your car!"

The effect of my words was simply amazing. What I saw then was like the denouement of an ancient Greek drama, a deus ex machina, where the gods suddenly swoop into the play, and miraculously, every problem is resolved. The corners of his lips softened and quivered as they began to levitate into a hesitant smile. His eyes widened as he began to rotate toward me. Looking at him, I saw his poor little Honda hatchback parked on Newberry Street—how it suffered dings and abuse from the Boston drivers who parked their cars in the murky slush. The drivers often parked by Braille, using their sense of touch to determine positioning as their bumpers slammed into the Honda's poor little chipped copper-colored painted body. I could envision him running outside on cold, wintry nights before 2:00 a.m. to move the car in compliance with the city's strict alternate side-of-the-street parking law to avoid a parking citation or, even worse, a visit from the tow truck. Then suddenly, he gasped and looked at me directly. His eyes were glazed over as though he was staring through me, focusing in the empty distance. I knew he was thinking about that fateful morning when he returned home after a night on call, seeking only peace and rest but instead finding his beloved Honda violated, the front passenger side window shattered, with broken glass strewn over the upholstery and adjacent street. And his car radio—an upgrade for which, as an addicted audiophile, he had paid for with money he did not have but managed to borrow—had been stolen. It was ripped mercilessly from the dashboard, with only a gaping hole and a loose tangle of wires remaining in its place, like a limb torn off on a bloody battlefield.

There was then a prolonged stillness, maybe thirty seconds or more, a moment of silence for the stricken, brave little car. I then heard a soft chuckle arise from deep in Terry's throat as his mind assessed the new possibilities. His entire face was smiling, with an open-mouthed, slightly asymmetric grin stretching from one huge blue glistening eye to the other. He pulled me close to him and now looked directly into my eyes. His lips grazed my ear and could feel my legs buckle as I heard him whisper, "What do you think about me moving in with you?"

I was amazed. I had often heard it said that the way to get a man to do what you want him to do is to make him think it is his idea, but I had never before actually seen it done. The use of this technique went against my feminist principles; it was an approach that was based upon deception and the puerile use of feminine wiles, but somehow, my feminist principles did not seem relevant at the moment. I looked at his luminous eyes, and before I melted into his kiss, I *innocently* murmured, "Oh? Oh! Gee…why not? Sounds good to me!"

Through his stomach? My ass. The way to a man's heart is clearly through his motorized vehicle.

At the time of my career meltdown, I was already in a committed relationship with Terry, who would eventually become my husband. I believe that this relationship, in fact, saved my life. When I decided to kill my dream, it was the personal happiness I had found with him that gave me the strength to choose a professional change rather than a personal tragic one. I was no longer going to be a doctor of Internal Medicine.

We had been living together for several months when I made the decision to leave my medical residency. I was disheveled emotionally. I had not conclusively determined what I would do, and whether or not I could still be any kind of physician, I was profoundly unhappy in mourning for my adolescent dreams, for my longstanding definition of self. I was not ready to present my conflict to Terry or to anybody, for that matter. And although the diagnostic possibilities I would consider would be considerably different if a patient presented to me with symptoms similar to mine, I erroneously assumed that the constant headaches, pins and needles, and intermittent blurry vision were due to stress. But the fact that I had determined what I did not want to do—in fact, what I *could* no longer do—brought about a peculiar sense of peace, belying the turmoil in my head.

The decision to become a radiologist was a decision that would necessitate starting, de novo, an entirely different course of postgraduate training. I would have to do another full residency. This decision was not reached lightly. I still wanted to be a doctor but realized that given my personal issues, to be really good at what I did, I needed to compartmentalize (i.e., limit my intense focus to the problem at hand to effectively evaluate a problem before becoming disabled by inexplicable fatigue). I was like a horse that needed blinders. I had to avoid being distracted by the myriad of extraneous medical and social issues that made a patient—a person. This was a task that could be, must be, successfully performed by practicing internists. My awareness that I could not effectively do this like others without excessive fatigue that resulted in the loss of focus, weakness, and physical collapse (why didn't I recognize the symptoms of MS?) was, to me, an admission of defeat. But alas, it had become clear that to do what was necessary to complete an evaluation in such a way as to satisfy my intense perfectionist nature without blowing my circuit breakers, I would have to undertake more focused tasks. I began to think of other specialties that would allow me to function in this way while still helping people, specialties that would still provide the intensity of intellectual challenge I continued to crave.

Over the next few weeks, I floated through the hospital departments in an attempt to find the answer. Dermatology? No, too focused…too limited in scope for my taste. Pathology? Intellectually challenging, but a specialty that to me seemed too removed from clinical issues. I'm not sure when the epiphany came but late in my second year of medical residency while managing a ward full of patients and continuing to supervise interns, I began to see a light at the end of the tunnel. I found a specialty that required a keen eye, highly trained interpretive skills, an encyclopedic knowledge with a rapid retrieval system, and the ability to provide accurate correlation with the clinical presentation. And all this was done quickly and succinctly, and…more importantly, with a clearly defined endpoint. The specialty required exquisite observation, and detection of findings, exceptionally educated evaluation and interpretation, and ultimate differential diagnosis and recommendations.

Next case, please.

I smiled. I had been told by my mother years before that stress does not come from working too hard. It comes from working hard while feeling as though you had no control of your own life…of your own destiny. I had found my salvation. I was going to be a radiologist. And I truly believed that I could be a very good one.

"Radiology?"

I couldn't tell if the soft but pained expression in Terry's voice represented disbelief, disappointment, disagreement, or just plain anger.

"You decided to go into the same field as me?"

His tone was increasingly annoyed.

"How did you make this decision? What were you thinking?"

His voice became louder.

"What about other fields, I don't know, Dermatology?"

His eyes were slits. He was pissed off. Terry and I were living together and had, in fact, become engaged to be married. Terry had gone through months of uncertainty about the logistics of marrying another physician. He had expressed concern about running a household and raising a family with two rather inflexible professions; however, I managed to convince him of my supernatural abilities to essentially become a professionally successful physician and June Cleaver—the wonder mom from the 1960s sitcom *Leave it To Beaver* wrapped into one. I actually had no idea how I would do this (I never could cook, for instance) or if it was in fact possible, yet I really wanted it to be true (and apparently so did Terry), so we both believed my fairy tale. I had now added the difficult logistics of finding two suitable and highly competitive career track positions in the same specialty and within the same geographic area. But I was determined to make this work, and in July of 1981, after completing two of the three years of my Internal Medicine residency at Tufts-New England Medical Center and only three months before my upcoming nuptials, I became a first-year Radiology resident at Harvard Medical School's Beth Israel Hospital in Boston.

I had never realized how fascinating diagnostic radiology was... nor did I realize how challenging [*sic*: down-right difficult] it could be. The ability to see true anatomic detail (as well as the secondary effects of nonvisualized structures on those you could see on plain radiographs) required a multitude of skills, many of which were never taught in medical school (such as the ability to visually extrapolate two-dimensional images to three) as well as skills you did learn in medical school (such as knowledge of the intricate interactive anatomy of all bodily structures) but to a degree of picayune detail you had never believed could be clinically relevant. But in diagnostic radiology, it was. A good radiologist had to be able to view a radiograph of any part of the body, quickly evaluate and subconsciously disregard the areas that fell into one of the innumerable variations of normal, and hone in on areas that could be considered any degree of abnormal (i.e., those which correlate with the patient's symptoms as well as those that do not [called incidental findings] that often reveal evidence of asymptomatic yet serious disease). The radiologist must be familiar with the physical and laboratory findings described by the clinicians, must understand the anatomy and physiology of disease states, and must have an encyclopedic knowledge of disease presentations and appearances—both common and exotic—to provide a differential diagnosis that can then be analyzed to provide for the correct diagnosis. And to add insult to injury, a radiologist in training is expected to understand the physics of radiology in exhaustive detail. If a film was not technically adequate for diagnostic assessment, we had to be able to recognize why and explain how to correct the problem. I finally saw a reason for physics in the required premedical college curriculum. As a college student, I had been so happy when I completed physics. I thought I was done with it for good. Wrong! When I became an intern and resident in internal medicine, we all believed that radiologists sat in dark rooms, drank coffee, and blandly read films. We would envy the *rads* for what we perceived as their separation from the dirty and intensely intellectual grind of clinical medicine as well as their more civilized lifestyles (i.e., we thought they were lazy technicians who were far removed from the arts and sciences of medicine, and although they earned incomes like [*sic*] real doctors they had a little true impact on patient care). As radiology residents, we learned how wrong these impressions were.

Our wedding was in the fall of my second year of training in radiology, and I had finally come to terms with the specialty and its relationship to my preconceived notion of a doctor. Although classically, radiologists had much less significant one-on-one contact with patients than did internists and surgeons, they were critical to the diagnosis of disease and often guided the appropriate evaluation and treatment of conditions, even some that would be otherwise unsuspected by the treating physician. A good radiologist had an enormous wealth of medical knowledge as well as finely tuned skills enabling him/her to detect and evaluate imaging findings and correlate these clinically. Although the actual recipient of this diagnostic acumen was the patient, the role of the radiologist was, in fact, that of a doctor's doctor—a consultant. I accepted this position understanding its value to the medical process, but my acceptance was always slightly ambivalent; it was subconsciously tinged with an element of regret at the loss of patient contact and with the need to recognize a new definition of a doctor. Terry never had a problem with this, which I presume was due to the fact that he chose his specialty in medical school when a student is just formulating his classification of the term physician and his perception of self within that depiction. At this point, he was a senior resident at MGH and was already a skilled radiologist; and after completion of his residency, he was planning to pursue subspecialty training in neuroradiology. Having already been accepted into the MGH neuroradiology fellowship program he was eagerly preparing to step into this fascinating yet complicated world. I could never detect a moment of doubt in him, which made an episode at our wedding even more poignant.

Just being a bride and dressing like a fairy princess at the age of twenty-nine years and six months (yes, my loving Jewish grandma, I made it before thirty!) was in itself an existential experience; the smiling face in the mirror, infused with impeccable yet subtle makeup and surrounded by a cascade of perfectly coifed blonde curls, was in fact mine. I could hardly recognize the happy, girlish young woman looking back at me from the glass, yet as I slowly walked down the aisle, all I could see was the beaming face of my husband-to-be, and I knew that this was really happening. As we stood under the lace and white rose-entwined wedding canopy with expectant, eager hearts, hand in hand, we faced the rabbi I had known since my childhood in Brooklyn. He smiled broadly and, while still gazing at me with what appeared to be almost paternal pride, began to speak.

"Oy vey! Is he okay?"

We all turned to see my elderly grandfather crumple to the floor. The rabbi was still speaking, now with an urgency I had previously only heard in his voice during Yom Kippur's sermons, "Is there a doctor in the house?" His voice trailed off as he realized the absurdity of his question.

In addition to the bride and groom, five additional members of the wedding party were young doctors although all of us were traveling incognito in white lace, tuxedos, and identical long lavender gowns with matching dyed satin shoes. The rabbi had barely finished his sentence as Terry and I dropped to our knees, and in complete disregard for the occasion and our formal attire, began to evaluate my grandfather, who was groggily awake.

"Grandpa…"

I gazed at the face of the small, frail man who had been a big, strong construction worker in years past and who, when I was a young child, would ignore the admonitions of my grandmother and as I shrieked with glee as he bounced me on his knee while still wearing his grimy work clothing. He would kiss me on the cheek, brushing my skin with his stubbly unshaven face, which, to his amusement, would cause me to complain that he was dusty. My grandfather made me feel special. He always smelled like cigars, infused with the aroma of cheap cherry tobacco that many people disdain but to this day, makes me feel loved and safe.

"Grandpa...," I softly continued with Terry close by my side. "We're doctors... Let us help you." We were checking his pulse and respirations when, although having barely recovered awareness, my grandfather, a hardworking and bluntly honest blue-collar immigrant and a man who always unconditionally loved me, grabbed my hand. While everyone waited expectantly for his words, his pale face, wrinkled by years of toil and suffering, seemed to droop further. I was his eldest grandchild, cherished granddaughter, and the first in his family to go to medical school; heck, the first to graduate from college. And it was my wedding day. I looked at the familiar bluish-gray eyes that had always glowed with hope for all five of his grandchildren, but which now appeared sunken, bloodshot, and watery. After slowly opening his mouth to speak, in a soft, barely audible voice, through pinched desiccated lips, he uttered with obvious disdain, "So what the hell'r you two gonna do? Take my picture?"

Another one with no respect for Radiology.

t takes a long time to become a radiologist. Back in the early 1980s, my era, most residencies started with a required one-year clinical internship followed by three years of radiology residency. The one-year internship was usually in either Internal Medicine or Surgery although some trainees elected to do an internship in which the fledgling doctor would switch services on a regular basis, known as a rotating internship. A rotating internship is less conducive to the development of specialized clinical expertise than would be a straight specialty internship. Doing a full straight residency in medicine or surgery encourages a strong identification with the specialty (i.e., *I am a surgeon* but switching to radiology after only one year in the specialty allows for the transition in self-definition to *I am a radiologist*). The young doctors who did a rotating internship did not appear to require a change in self-definition; they seemed to consider themselves radiologists from the beginning. They were aware that clinical internship training was a necessary part of their denouement and of their radiological evolution. For them, the internship offered an insight into the problems encountered by several specialties as they relate to medical imaging, possibly making them better radiologists. I completed two years of a straight Internal Medicine residency before switching to radiology, and because of this had already begun to think of myself as an internist.

The process of considering myself a radiologist seemed to require a longer period of evolution than most. Actually, I'm not certain that it was ever really complete. Radiology is a medical science in which imaging and the accuracy of its interpretation are used as a window into the complex anatomy and physiology of the human body. It enables the radiologist to differentiate wellness from illness and gives him hard data which, when accurately interpreted, allows him to further categorize illness in mind-boggling detail. The radiologist is a physician who provides diagnostic information to the physician who is directly caring for the patient and, by doing so, provides a critical service to the patient and to his doctor. Internal medicine is different. Sure, an educated evaluation of objective findings within the history, physical exam, and laboratory data is necessary for accurate diagnosis of disease, but in patient care, it is not everything. Not by a long shot. Somehow, I could still hear my medicine professors preaching about how in addition to considering the physical findings and laboratory data, a doctor needs to look at the patient and listen to him for the intangible, subjective findings which can provide priceless insight into the patient himself, offering great assistance in the evaluation of his illness. We were taught that knowing the patient as well as his disease is critical if one is to provide optimal care. This is the part of practicing medicine that is an art. This is the part I was going to miss.

I became pregnant with our first child while working as a senior resident in radiology. Although it would be romantic to say that our son was unintentionally conceived during an episode of passionate and reckless abandon, it is more accurate to say that his creation was the product of vigilant planning and timing. It appeared that for a woman, the senior year of her radiology residency was the optimal time to initiate gestation; she could drastically limit her radiation exposure by performing professorial delegation of duty to the more junior residents, a custom that was universally instituted and universally resented by the junior trainees.

The practice of senior residency pregnancy was so ubiquitous that it spawned many inside jokes. For example, to become board certified in Diagnostic Radiology by the American Board of Radiology, the resident must take a grueling examination known as the Boards. The initial part of this fearsome assessment is a written test given during the course of the residency, which determines competency in clinical and scientific (ugh, physics!) knowledge. Although quite challenging, by this time in our educational careers, we were very familiar with the curriculum we were expected to have mastered. Armed with number 2 pencils, our extensive education, and the knowledge of how to accurately color the bubble next to the correct answer, we were undaunted. In short, we could readily handle whatever written test the board chose to put in front of us, completing the task while comfortable in our physical (and metaphysical) anonymity.

In contrast to this, the second and final part of the national boards in Diagnostic Radiology was a very personal, oral examination given in June just prior to the completion of residency. For this, all the senior radiology residents in the country were required to fly to Louisville, Kentucky, in early June (and it was not to attend the derby which is held in May).

Instead, at one infamous hotel adorned with rich, thick, velvet-patterned paper adorning walls in a different deep royal hue in every room (much like a nineteenth-century bordello), we presented ourselves, individually and alone, for the practical examination. We were each given a list of world-renowned professors assigned to us, as well as schedule. Each professor was a published expert in their focused subspecialty within radiology.

At the ringing of a bell, we would walk into the first room, where the illustrious doctor (whose name was more famous to us than Mick Jagger) would sometimes utter a polite hello while holding a stack of radiographs. Often, the professor would say absolutely nothing, would hang the films on a view box one at a time, and would sit back, expecting the young doctor to start talking. We were expected to evaluate and interpret, suggest the clinical presentation, differentially diagnose and recommend therapy or any additional studies if needed.

The examiner would then ask, "Are you finished?"

And if you answered in the affirmative, would take the film down and put up the next. Sometimes this would be the follow-up study you suggested (*hallelujah!*), sometimes, it would be a different follow-up study, and sometimes, it would simply be the next unrelated case. You would never be told if you were accurate, nor did you ever know for sure. After a suitable time interval, a bell would ring, and you would leave the room of the stony-faced professor and head to your next examination to be performed by another world-famous radiologist who similarly tortured you within his or her area of renowned expertise. This would continue relentlessly until you were tested in all the areas deemed important to the practice of radiology by the American Board of Radiology, and when you were done, you had no idea how well or poorly you had performed and whether or not you had passed until about a week later when you were back at your residency program. Nobody uttered a word about the experience for fear of appearing (or actually discovering you were) inadequate and had completely missed the boat. The feeling was similar to the one associated with a recurring nightmare each of us had during our college years, which I have since learned is a symptom of an obsessive personality, about facing a final exam in a class for which we were completely unprepared and in which we didn't previously realize we were enrolled. Eventually, one would be called individually into the chairman's office for the reading of the verdict. I never heard of a resident having a heart attack during this time, but I would not be surprised if it has happened.

Obviously, the experience of the oral boards was a critical, stressful time in the life of a senior radiology resident, and thus, it generated a great deal of folklore regarding improving the likelihood of a victorious outcome. This was the early 1980s when the concept of dress for success was becoming popular, providing fodder for many magazine articles and how-to books for the twentysomethings (and some early thirtysomethings following prolonged medical training) about to enter the business and professional worlds. Therefore, most of us believed that a male senior resident should present himself in a professional manner. Although an outfit of green scrubs was de rigueur for working in the hospital, this was unacceptable for his appearance for the oral exam at the Louisville bordello. It was generally agreed that he should wear a long-sleeve solid color (preferably white or blue) business shirt and tie, black dress shoes, black socks, all framing a dark suit or sports jacket, and dress slacks (dark blues and grays are fine, but for some reason, never brown). And, of *course*, a matching belt.

The appropriate outfit for a female senior resident was more complicated and generated a great deal of discussion and disagreement. Although the young woman physician wanted to look professional and thus be taken seriously by the examiner, there was the danger of appearing too masculine, and by doing so, risk disturbing the subconscious sensibilities of the, at that time, largely male group of examiners. Therefore, we discussed appropriate attire with an attention to detail, befitting our necessary nit-picking profession. We debated about fitted versus unfitted jackets, padded versus flat shoulders, cotton versus silk blouses, and pants versus skirts, with endless discussions about skirt length, pantyhose (yes or no), and the preferred height of the heel of the sensible yet feminine leather pumps. The arguments were infinite, and the various opinions were all well substantiated. Finally, amazingly, we reached an agreement. We decided to be sensible. It was determined that the appropriate outfit to be worn by a female senior radiology resident to the oral boards was…a maternity dress. And it was practical too.

I felt great during my pregnancy. I'd heard all the stories about morning sickness, water retention, insomnia, urinary frequency, constipation, and the like. I guess I had some of these symptoms, but overall, I felt really good, especially in the second trimester. I joked that in the first trimester a pregnant woman looks fat instead of *heavy with child*. In the second trimester, the excuse for her constant complaining is finally evident, but the condition is still not as physically cumbersome as in the third trimester when she becomes really big when the stranger developing within essentially takes dominion over her body. I could joke about pregnancy because, in general, I felt better through all three trimesters than I had in years. It was later that I learned that the heavy hormonal load of pregnancy actually puts multiple sclerosis into a kind of remission.

After my residency was over and I had successfully (thank God!) completed the Diagnostic Radiology boards, it was time to consider practicing my trade. It was July in Boston, and it was very hot and humid. I had always felt awful in the heat; for example, I could never enjoy a summer day basking in the sun at the beach, which I later realized was because of my MS. Apparently, nerve conduction is always slowed by heat. People with normal nervous systems are often not aware of this, which I suspect is because the effective slowing caused by warm weather or hot water does not drop their nerve conduction below a critical threshold for symptoms. Those of us with MS, however—whose nerve conductivity is already standing on a banana peel—are dramatically more symptomatic under warmer conditions. We are always at or below this critical threshold, and heat simply throws us under the bus. Obviously, hot weather makes MS sufferers feel lousy, but during the summer of 1984, I felt worse than I had in earlier summers likely due to my advanced state of pregnancy. In fact, it was easy to blame the pregnancy for all my symptoms. My child was due in September, and Terry's fellowship in Neuroradiology would not be over until January, at which time we could both seek employment. Although being seven or eight months pregnant was uncomfortable, pregnancy was not something I considered a job, and I would lose my mind just sitting around the apartment. It was a one-bedroom condo, so I had no baby's room to decorate, and it was just too hot outside to lug my belly around doing other activities. I could no longer, whenever I felt the urge, shop at Filene's Basement, which I considered the original off-priced store. I loved that place, especially back in the 1980s when it was the real deal, and you could follow wonderful designer merchandise until it was marked down to a ridiculously low price.

No…instead, I responsibly sought temporary employment as a radiologist. I wanted to do a locum tenens, which is a fancy term used by professionals to obscure its true meaning. In fact, I was looking for a job as a *temp*. While Terry's life was engulfed by the high-intensity, groundbreaking academic and clinical world of neuroradiology at Massachusetts General Hospital, I found a temporary position practicing general community radiology with a hospital group in the northern suburbs of Boston, allowing the regular group members to take summer vacations. I could work without the stresses of long hours, night calls, or running a practice. The other radiologists were happy to have me there, and as a temporary employee, I cost them a lot less than another full-time associate—a win-win. It was a lovely existence, and I was happily employed until my stress-free life came to a screeching halt. It was a few days before my due date, and the symptoms of labor were impossible to misinterpret.

As any mother will attest, the birth of a first child is an experience like no other.

Participating, particularly for the first time, in the arrival of a tiny human being who is actually part of both you and the man you love is existential in its beauty and is actually somewhat surreal.

Labor and delivery, however, are not. It appears that women psychologically block out the painful experience of childbirth. We remember the intense joy of having a baby, but the rest is a cognitive blur. This is fortunate for all subsequent children. If we really remembered what it was like, every first child would also be the last.

I was admitted to Boston's Beth Israel Hospital. This was the same hospital in which I did my radiology residency, so in addition to having outstanding attending physicians, labor and delivery nurses, and obstetrical facilities, it was also replete with resident physicians, albeit junior to me, many of whom I knew well during my training. However, I was now a patient and was supposed to be treated as such, and the ob-gyn residents directly responsible for my care were appropriately skilled, professional, and courteous. But there was the one male surgical resident who ran into my room during a peak contraction and, with a feigned expression of clinical concern, shoved a radiograph directly in front of my gasping face and asked for my professional radiological opinion. After the contraction abated, I gave him my opinion, but I must say that it was not related to the film he was holding, nor was it very professional. He just laughed. Thinking back, I remembered that he had been a lowly surgical intern during my senior year of radiology residency, at which time he was not very good at assessing a routine emergency room x-ray. On a Monday morning during his internship, after he had gone through a particularly harrowing Sunday night of call, he came to the radiology department. Unwashed and disheveled, bearing bloodshot eyes and wearing swamp water green scrubs stained with blood and other unidentifiable body fluids, he politely asked me to review with him films taken on patients he admitted during the night. Perhaps I (who, as a senior resident, was well-slept, bathed, and refreshed) had interpreted some of his studies. While seated comfortably in my overstuffed burgundy leather chair, I described the findings in unnecessary and condescending detail. I probably displayed a supercilious look which, although unwittingly, expressed a low opinion of the intern's abilities.

Oh well, sorry. Insensitive. Hey, I had been an intern too, buddy, and I lived through the abuse. You know, *it ain't easy being queen.* I guess sometimes I was the jerk. And for this highly trained and capable senior surgical resident, this was sweet revenge!

As any new mother will confirm, the birth of a first baby is never what one expects. The two nights in the hospital, where the baby sleeps elsewhere and is presented only when he happily needs cuddling or nursing, is essentially a vacation in Hawaii. Although I believed that my maternal fortitude was tested and confirmed by acceptance of the gentle awakening by a nurse at 2:00 a.m. to feed a hungry, bathed, and diapered infant, the reality of the situation about to be experienced upon discharge bore no resemblance to the hospital coddling. Terry and I took our baby son home to our one-bedroom high-rise apartment in downtown Boston in our neon-colored orangey-copper Honda Accord two-door hatchback, which required yoga-like contortions and athletic agility to properly insert the infant car seat. And it was even harder to insert the infant. The baby did not understand what we were doing, was unaware of (and did not care about) our inexperience, and was generally uncooperative. Despite all the books and videos (not to mention our intense medical education, including pediatric clinical rotations), we were well-intentioned but clueless. We were new, first-time parents.

After the birth of the baby in September 1984, I stopped working to take care of our infant and apartment full-time. I was biding time until January, at which point Terry would have completed his Neuroradiology fellowship, and the two of us could search the country in earnest together for permanent positions: his in neuroradiology and mine in general radiological practice. So for the time being, I was a full-time housewife and mother. How hard could it be? High school dropouts did it all the time, apparently successfully. For a few weeks, I was generally disoriented. I remember awakening from a deep sleep at 2:00 a.m. on the first night home, wondering where the wailing cat was, until I realized that instead of the squeals of a distraught kitten in the dark city streets, the high-pitched cries I was hearing belonged to my newborn son requesting feeding and changing. And unfortunately for me as a nursing mother, no matter what the hour, feeding was my responsibility. Although I am aware of all the scientific studies describing the benefits that breastfeeding offers both the child and the mother, I couldn't help but suspect that the whole concept was a male conspiracy created to ensure their restful sleep.

Keeping up with the infant's incessant needs and demands could be a full-time job in itself. It was time to organize a system. And after a few fitful weeks, I had it figured out. I had designed a schedule that included full child care allowing for general maternal sustenance, including showering and dressing myself, eating, and preparing dinner for my new little family. Of course, there was also the occasional excursion for grocery shopping, taken on foot with baby in tow (we lived in downtown Boston and driving would be akin to suicide), performed by securely attaching my child to the front of my body with a simple yet overpriced, powder blue, papoose-like canvas strap. This was a device used by all the professional women I knew who were also currently masquerading as mothers and who purchased all the latest parenting tools, which in addition to keeping the baby secure, ensured that he would soil his diaper as soon as we were ready to leave, assuring the need to start the preparation process all over. It was a challenging job at best. And although I had the entire daily regimen as virtually well-orchestrated and rehearsed as the workup of a chest pain patient admitted through the emergency room, it was rare that I was ever able to achieve anything even closely successful.

Although I felt surprisingly well during pregnancy, after the baby was born, I was overcome with indescribable fatigue. Treatment for the usual postpartum anemia offered little relief. It was a tiredness that I could not easily describe, one that no amount of rest or sleep could help, one that perhaps only death would relieve. It was the kind of fatigue that I later learned was common in multiple sclerosis and that the hormones of pregnancy were helpful in minimizing this as well as other symptoms of MS, which would suddenly rebound after delivery and drop in the hormones. My legs became heavy weights, and although the symptoms were subtle, my hands were less functional for detailed fine-motor tasks. And hot showers—anathema to people with MS—made all my symptoms worse. On many evenings, Terry would come home from the hospital to find the baby well cared for, but the apartment was unkempt. His wife, who had formerly demonstrated something akin to a superwoman existence, had not yet showered, was still in pajamas, and was very, very tired.

I struggled by. I had to; my baby depended on me, and my husband believed he had a wife. I noticed that my hand symptoms progressed, experiencing extreme numbness of my thumb and adjacent two fingers; a region of the hand described in medical jargon as a radial distribution, which means on the thumb side of the hand that corresponds to the location of the radius bone in the forearm. This part of the hand receives sensory nerve impulses (which are necessary to feel things) from the median nerve. I saw several doctors for my symptoms and eventually received a diagnosis of carpal tunnel syndrome: a condition in which the soft tissue tunnel in the wrist through which the median nerve passes is somehow compressing the nerve and compromising its function. This is a condition often seen in people who repeatedly traumatize the area by overuse (i.e., typists, pianists, jackhammer operators, etc.).

It was pointed out to me, however, that pregnancy commonly triggers the condition due to fluid retention and swelling of the tissues of the carpal tunnel. Although this seemed to make sense as I had recently been pregnant, it did not explain why I had no symptoms during pregnancy, with the numbness spontaneously appearing after the delivery of my baby. While the actual timing was not characteristic of carpal tunnel syndrome, it was, in fact, consistent with a flare of multiple sclerosis after childbirth, where the sudden drop in pregnancy hormones triggers inflammation in the central nerves of the brain or spinal cord, which in turn results in diminished signals to the peripheral sensory nerves which innervate the thumb side of the hand. This timing issue was not appreciated at the time. I was sent for nerve conduction studies designed to evaluate the level of neurological dysfunction. It turns out that the results of the test were, in fact, indeterminate and not clearly consistent with carpal tunnel syndrome. I was therefore referred to a hand surgeon for further evaluation and consideration of operative release of the presumed offending carpal tunnel soft tissue band. The hand surgeon was a renowned surgical professor and was probably considered the best hand surgeon in Boston, which in this medical town was quite an honor. His supercilious haughtiness was consistent with his level of prestige. After examining me, he quickly glanced at my chart, scanned the results of my nerve study, and, with a sharp flick of the wrist, tossed my chart into the hands of the surgical scheduling nurse who was succinctly presenting my history. Upon hearing that my husband was a neuroradiology fellow, he turned to me and sneered.

"Well then, why are you coming to me," his voice clearly demeaning, "a mere surgeon for diagnosis and treatment of your nerve problem, Doc? Can't your husband simply image your nerve?" He turned and chuckled with his fellows, who dutifully laughed with him. They were board-certified orthopedic surgeons who were undergoing advanced training with the master in a hand-surgery fellowship and dutifully followed his every word. I hung my head, both in shame and deference, and a few days later underwent surgery for a carpal tunnel release. As it turns out, I did not need the surgery. The reason my nerve-conduction studies did not clearly demonstrate carpal tunnel syndrome was because I did not have carpal tunnel syndrome. My symptoms were due to the fluctuating neurological impairment of multiple sclerosis, and although I felt better as expected six weeks after my surgery, the resolution of my symptoms was also consistent with the relapsing-remitting nature of my MS at the time. I have since had an interesting thought about my initial encounter with the hand surgeon. Although I admit that MRI (magnetic resonance imaging) was not a clinically available tool at the time, today, MRI is a powerful technique used by neuroradiologists for the diagnosis of disorders of the central nervous system. If it had been available when I saw the hand surgeon, an MRI of my brain would have accurately revealed the cause of my symptoms by demonstrating the imaging findings, now considered diagnostic, of multiple sclerosis—a diagnosis that was also consistent with the results of my confusing nerve-conduction studies. So yes, famous doctor, sir, as you so sarcastically asked me, my husband can now essentially image my nervous system and, as you incorrectly attempted years ago, determine the cause of my symptoms.

The only difference is, sir, his diagnosis would have been correct.

I n February 1985, I joined a hospital-based practice, which staffed two hospitals west of Fort Lauderdale. We lived in a carpeted two-bedroom, two-bathroom, two-story rented townhouse with a dishwasher, washer, and dryer in a middle-class community located northwest of Fort Lauderdale. It was painted a basic off-white, with scattered plugs of white spackle, providing firm confirmation of a previous tenant. There was new clean beige standard-issue, stain-resistant, flat-textured carpeting laid over the thinnest padding known to man, providing confirmation of our presence as a new tenant. Inexpensive framed posters interspersed with our framed diplomas tastefully adorned the living room walls and the standard cozy (small) rectangular rooms lovingly decorated with hand-me-down furniture, supplemented by a few accent pieces from Pier One. There were sliding glass doors (on which we put stickers to prevent our crashing into them), which opened onto a minuscule cement patio and a man-made lake. This, in reality, was a tiny pond, replete with insects and hungry, dirty ducks who would squawk all night. But unlike our one-bedroom, twenty-third-story apartment in Boston, to us, this was a suburban dream home. We now had two bedrooms, which meant that, unlike in Boston, the baby had his own room! As the only room in the house adorned with new furniture (donations from relatives), crib bedding, mobiles, and wall decorations (gifts from friends), it was happiness in blue, with a ceiling painted like a morning sky dusted with sunshine and cloudy wisps of white-painted as part of an artistic project which celebrated a rare family weekend off together. When my beeper went off at night and I had to get out of bed, wash the fatigue from my eyes, and drive to the hospital to manage an emergency, it was my baby's beaming face—and his angelic room—that gave me strength.

Our existence was pretty tumultuous, and free time was nonexistent. I was always completely exhausted, but this raised no suspicions in that it was easily explained by my insane schedule or, in reality, by the lack thereof. Life was like a canoe of overwhelming responsibility floating in completely unpredictable waters...and something was always rocking the boat. It was less than five minutes from one of my hospitals—the one at which I was usually assigned during the day although, at night and on weekends, I also covered another hospital over twenty miles away. I received full-time help with the baby from a lovely middle-aged woman who came to my house every morning and who left every evening when I returned. But when I came home, I was a full-time wife and mommy. I made dinner (poorly) almost every night, cleaned up, and tended to my son and husband. Terry's practice was demanding, with night-call and frequent weekends at the hospital, but so was mine! We tried to stagger our call schedules so that someone would always be available for the baby in the evenings and on weekends. My husband and I probably did not spend enough time on the relationship necessary to maintain healthy communication although we obviously communicated somewhat. When the baby turned twelve months of age, I became pregnant again.

During my second pregnancy, I was no longer a senior radiology resident but instead was a hospital-based radiologist in private practice and not yet a partner in the group. I realized that I had reached a critical point in my career; an intersection where the electricity was interrupted, and traffic lights were flashing yellow in four directions. The way I handled my pregnancy and practice could determine my long-term success...or failure. My concern dated back to the days in which I first sought employment. Most radiology groups, at least those in South Florida, were comprised only of men. At that time, many radiology groups were afraid to hire young women radiologists because of their fear that the woman would decrease her workload during pregnancy, which would require the other doctors to work harder in order to pick up the slack. Having assured the other doctors in my group that this would not be a problem, I now had to prove it. I was expected to handle my share of the work without special consideration, and it was very important to everyone that I fulfill the promise I made. So I continued working full-time, did all the requested procedures, wore heavy lead aprons, and took full night call. Surprisingly, after the first few months of morning sickness, I was able to function well, readily juggling the roles of practice and motherhood. It was not until my second baby was born that I again started to unravel.

Shortly after childbirth, the indescribable fatigue would frequently grip my body. It was as though I was a swimmer caught in a rip current, an irresistible force dragging me under the water and tearing me away from my life. The strength in my upper legs, arms, and hands would episodically wane. The symptoms were nonspecific enough to be readily blamed on lack of sleep or on the frequent lifting of an infant and a toddler. I now realize that, while pregnant, I experienced (as during my first pregnancy) a dramatic remission of many of my MS symptoms, then developing what a severe flair following delivery was. This is a classic scenario for multiple sclerosis. Apparently, the amazing wisdom of Mother Nature provides a type of immune suppression to a pregnant mother to allow her fetus (who is genetically foreign to the mother with half of its DNA from the father) to develop unimpeded, without the mom's natural immunity mounting a rejection response toward her developing child. In a woman with multiple sclerosis, there is the added bonus of this natural magic, providing suppression of the mom's wacky immune system, markedly decreasing her body's tendency to destroy her own nervous system. This immune suppression dramatically drops after delivery, which often frequently triggers a severe exacerbation of MS. My medical judgment (as well as that of colleagues treating my symptoms) was again markedly clouded by denial. I even had a flair-up of my pseudo–carpal tunnel syndrome following childbirth (this time in the opposite hand, which compounded the misdiagnosis) and underwent a second real surgery for misdiagnosed carpal tunnel release.

Ah, Mother Nature…how does a girl get some of your magic potion?

I continued to work as a radiologist, practicing as part of a hospital-based group that provided Radiology coverage for two hospitals 24-7, not an uncommon arrangement. This required, from each doctor, forty-five to fifty hours per week of intense work in either of the two hospitals, which were each over twenty miles from my home. In addition to these hours, each radiologist provided a full week each month of additional required "coverage," (i.e., performing and interpreting exams at night and on the weekend) This was before the days of computer-based images viewable from home, so the *on-call* radiologist would drive to and from both hospitals—often several times a night—only to return the next day for a regular day of work. One year, I noticed that I put over fifty thousand miles on my car's odometer.

So I was fatigued. Big surprise. But…I did lots of breast imaging. I found that I loved interpreting mammograms while other radiologists apparently did not. I often found the difficult cases piled in my stack, and I was happy to interpret them—a *win-win*, so to speak. In the 1980s, my Radiology residency program in Boston was very strong in breast imaging, which at the time consisted largely of mammography. I was taught by clinical professors who really loved it. They told us they were motivated by the belief that mammography was an unusually *proactive* component of medicine (i.e., instead of diagnosing illness and injury after the fact, lives could potentially be saved by identifying a worrisome finding before it was clinically evident, often well before it could become a life-threatening problem). The excitement felt by my professors was contagious; so much so that I welcomed the more challenging and difficult breast cases. Although this excitement followed me into practice, my schedule had become inconsistent with the life I wanted. My boys were very young, and I felt that I couldn't focus on them at all. Even when I was home, I was completely exhausted and needy. Instead of seeing a mother, my children saw a frazzled woman who lived there a few hours a week. They were being raised by nannies, and despite the job satisfaction I felt by embarking upon a full-fledged career, I felt that I had to make a change, at least for the time being. So in an outpatient center close to home, I found a job that was not on a partnership track.

Although I worked forty-five hours a week, it was considered part-time in that it required no night or weekend calls, and there was a lot of mammography. It provided everything I needed as a professional *working mom*, and although the pay was significantly lower than that of a partner, it was by no means terrible. I continued to have occasional episodes of weakness, dizziness, and fatigue, but what working mom does not feel overworked?

So why did I leave the outpatient diagnostic radiology office? What was missing? Was it the money? The glory? The *second-class* status presumed by other doctors? In all honesty, I cannot be sure that these were not contributing factors. But there was something else wrong. I could not figure out what that was although the frequent neurological symptoms certainly contributed. I needed to fix things, both for myself and my family.

Instead of admitting that something was in fact wrong with *me*, as a defense mechanism, a supercilious sense of superiority took over. What I needed was to find a practice that would highlight my skills within a narrow area of focus.

Breast imaging quickly came to mind. It was an area of radiology for which I had gotten a good deal of training during my residency. One of my professors there was a pioneer in breast imaging and truly loved to teach. In my earlier full-time practices, I often found the difficult mammograms tossed upon my pile of cases to read, as everybody knew that I didn't mind. Breast imaging seemed like a good choice. And to be honest, I was so tired. I could not continue the full-time practice of diagnostic radiology, which could be physically demanding. I was still in my thirties, but I felt like I was eighty. So I quit the full-time practice. Again, I had to ignore the overwhelming feeling of failure that welled up inside of me. I had to present a front to my children and my husband, and I began working at a mammography office run by private enterprise. I would just work about three and a half days a week in four-hour sessions. I was more aggressive than the radiologists they had before, which initially caused some problems. I recommended biopsies far more frequently than they were used to, which was upsetting to them and to their patients. I was called in for many discussions with the administration. After about six months, they stopped complaining…as they discovered that I was finding a large number of cancers at an early curable stage.

I worked at this practice for a few years. Although it was far less satisfying than what I wanted, it provided a time where I could regroup, feel less fatigued, and…have a third baby! I was thirty-eight years old when I became pregnant. It was certainly going to be the last baby. Since I already had two boys, I would be dishonest if I said I wasn't hoping for a girl.

I worked throughout the pregnancy, and although I found the physiological changes of pregnancy were less well-tolerated by my older body, there was a notable improvement in my overall sense of well-being. Once again, I felt better during pregnancy, not unusual in multiple sclerosis. My beautiful daughter was born on a dazzlingly sunny and breezy day in May, one month after my thirty-ninth birthday.

I was able to spend more time with my children and with my family; however, there was still something wrong. It was probably in part related to intermittent symptoms of multiple sclerosis. However, a large part of my ennui was due to the fact that I missed the heart of medicine that I loved—the part that made me become a doctor in the first place. I wanted to see patients again. I had not totally recovered from my exodus from internal medicine, and I wanted to speak with, listen to, and examine patients.

A breast center—a clinically oriented center with imaging, patient interaction with physical exam, as well as diagnostic procedures. I told myself that this was the way to hone in on my excellence, limiting my medical attention to one area that I knew completely. This made sense to me without damaging my ego. I did not recognize at the time that I was also establishing a way to limit my practice of medicine to a level that I (with my compromised immune system, intermittent inexplicable physical symptoms, and sporadic overwhelming fatigue) could endure without the entire structure of my self-esteem toppling down. So on October 18, 1993, with the business support of my husband and financial support of a bank, I opened the Center for Mammography and Breast Diagnostics.

The office was everything I could hope for. Unlike most radiologists, I would see and examine every patient. I would talk to them and advise them, allowing for the satisfaction of the internist still within me. A technician would perform a mammogram that I would interpret on-site. If extra views were needed, they would be done immediately, avoiding the panic felt by women from a callback. I would perform a physical exam on every patient, and if indicated by a finding on the mammogram or from my breast exam, I myself would perform a breast ultrasound on the patient without missing a beat, making it seem like a routine part of the evaluation. I would be talking with the women about anything on their minds—both medical and social—nonstop throughout the visit. This girl talk allowed for distraction from what I was doing, thereby avoiding the patient's understandable panic of knowing that more views or ultrasound were needed. If a biopsy was then needed, I could explain it like a friend and schedule the patient for an image-guided biopsy also to be performed by me. No special referrals. An unsuspected advantage of this type of practice allowed me to discuss and counsel patients about many other problems about which they were troubled. They were comfortable talking with me.

I loved this practice. Although the reason for my job satisfaction was not entirely obvious to me at the time, it certainly is now. Although I was a radiologist providing imaging studies and interpretation, unlike most radiologists, I had a great deal of face-time with my patients. They would tell me their medical problems, I would clinically and radiologically evaluate them, and I would discuss the findings and my recommendations directly with them. I did not have to tell another doctor, who would then tell the patients what I found and what I suggested. There would always be something intangible lost in the retelling. Nobody could provide the patient with the care related to her visit like I could, and I loved it. For me, it had a real but intrinsically limited (thus manageable) aspect of internal medicine.

In a world where radiologists are specialists who provide information to primary care doctors in order to assist them in the care of patients with whom they had direct contact, I had become a logical inconsistency—a primary-care radiologist!

My practice became wildly successful. I loved it. Patients loved it too! They were thrilled to be evaluated in this way, and I quickly established a system whereby I saw patients four days a week, leaving the fifth day for performing stereotactic (X-ray-guided) and ultrasound-guided core needle biopsies, leaving some open time as well for the frequent add-on patients referred by their doctors who needed immediate evaluation. I was finding cancers that were not identified on screening mammograms but could be felt by either the patients or by me on physical examination. I would identify metastases (or the spread of a known cancer) by performing a lymph node examination. This would allow the patient to be evaluated and treated by a surgeon and/or an oncologist (cancer specialist) without delay, which could improve the likelihood of a good outcome. I became so busy that I was booked very far in advance. It was difficult to get an appointment with me such that I could no longer accept new patients. This resulted in people using tricks to be seen by me. Although there were many other techniques used, most would ask their doctor to refer them as an emergency. Amusingly, I received a telephone call from my sister-in-law in Philadelphia. A friend of hers (who lived in Pennsylvania but who wintered in Florida) noticed that we both had the same last name, made the connection, and had her call me on her behalf! I must admit—that one worked.

Throughout the 1990s, I was having frequent symptoms that should have alerted either me or my husband to a significant neurologic condition. If either of us had seen a patient with my signs and symptoms, we would have suspected the diagnosis. I guess that when you or your spouse is the one experiencing the symptoms and showing the signs...well...denial is certainly a powerful coping mechanism.

Eventually, my disease grabbed us by the collar and shook us awake.

I t was December 2000, and we were in Long Island, New York. We were in a hotel room, getting ready for my young cousin's lush, fairy-tale wedding when (as married couples occasionally do) we engaged in a heated discussion about something or other and—

I do not remember the reason we argued, but I will never forget the ferocious and frightening feelings that suddenly enveloped me; the essential paralysis of my right side, the inability to form words with my mouth, and a sudden visual haziness. My body and mind were possessed by an alien force.

We flew home the next day. We hardly said a word to each other on the plane. I'm not sure what he was thinking. However, my mind was searching the past, uncovering episodes that were certainly indications of my neurologic disease although not detected by myself or my husband. I have to say if I saw you with my symptoms, I would have at least suspected the neurologic problem. I started to feel embarrassed about my lack of clinical acumen. I remember the time when my family went to England. My sons were fourteen and twelve, and my daughter was seven. We were taking long walks to different tourist sites, and I could hardly keep up. My little daughter was faster than me. Elderly folks, while engrossed in conversation, readily passed me by. Later in the afternoon, as my family and other tourists eagerly scrambled up onto a tour bus, I caused a significant delay as I could hardly lift my leg onto the first step. The driver kindly hauled me onto the bus, and several people offered me their seats. My family either did not notice or would not acknowledge the peculiar scene. Oh my god, what were we thinking? My children were young and probably didn't understand. However, my husband and I seemed to be experiencing the same denial.

The morning after we returned from the Long Island wedding, I was scheduled for an MRI of my brain. This was long after the trip to England—magnetic resonance imaging. Although I had never had one before, the technology was not new to me. My goodness, I am a radiologist. I knew all about the modality. I knew that I'd be lying on a moving table with my head and neck locked in a vice. I knew that I'd have something injected into a vein, and then the table would move me into an enclosed, coffin-like space where I'd stay for over an hour. I knew that I'd be wearing noise-canceling headphones that supplied soothing music, which failed to cancel the incessant *boom-boom-boom* of the machine. I knew it was safe. No radiation. Only strong magnets. Just magnets. But I also knew the possible diagnoses we'd be looking for. An MRI...

On the day of the study, I awakened in a free-floating panic. I couldn't draw air into my lungs. My diaphragm would not work without conscious effort. I had experienced this feeling before, but now my armpits and eyes seemed to liquefy, my throat constricting.

My husband, the neuroradiologist, performed the procedure. I could tell that he was nervous too. The differential diagnoses for my array of symptoms included very ominous conditions, including a stroke, unusual infection...or a brain tumor. Our well-organized, highly functional, long-lived defense mechanism was coming apart. It was very clear that I had a neurological problem. Our eyes had been forced open, and the walls of our communal denial came tumbling down. He came into the exam room, immediately following the procedure and was smiling a weird smile I had never seen before on the lips of my husband of twenty years.

"Good news!" he announced. "You have multiple sclerosis!"

I smiled too. The intrinsic irony of our relief was palpable. I didn't have a brain tumor.

Now that I had a diagnosis, I had many decisions to make. Do I tell my office staff? Do I discuss it with my young children? Do I tell anybody? I answered no to all these questions. I could still work. The disease did not yet affect my vision, ability to think, or the sensitivity of my hands and fingers. My ability to identify abnormalities on mammograms and logically assess and evaluate was intact. I could talk to patients, perform stereotactic biopsies, and use an ultrasound probe for both diagnosis and biopsy guidance. My symptoms were intermittent. Fortunately, as my own boss, I could adjust my schedule around my flairs so as not to affect my ability to provide the best patient care. As I did not intend to close my office, I didn't want my employees to worry and look for other jobs.

I certainly didn't want to upset my children, so I acted as though everything was normal. In this regard, I was only fooling myself. Even the youngest of children are aware of something wrong with their mother. They were already worried. Retrospectively, I think I should have explained something to them so as to ease their anxiety. Talking about it, however, would increase my anxiety. I guess I made my decision mostly based on concern about myself—the fear of losing my identity.

Awareness of my illness would be on a *need-to-know* basis.

I saw a neurologist and began what would be years of therapy, starting with a medication that required refrigeration that I injected into my thigh daily. I continued to work. I was careful to reschedule patients when I wasn't right. When this was the case, usually, it meant difficulties with my gait or problems related to my urinary and digestive system. I was not experiencing fluctuations in my vision, finger sensitivity, or cognitive abilities to any significant degree, symptoms that could impair my ability to function at a high level. There were days when I went from room to room while leaning on the wall.

As I explained, a good portion of my work involved talking to people, learning about their medical problems as well as the psychosocial issues causing them pain. An important reason women came to see me was to unburden themselves to a nonjudgmental authority figure—a girlfriend analog but one who could provide educated as well as caring dialogue. There was a desperate yearning for advice with no topics unacceptable and without the need for political correctness. I was able to suppress the occasionally nagging feeling that my problems were worse than theirs. I would remind myself that no matter how many people are in our lives, we are each a lonely ballerina pirouetting on the stage of existence. As a result, to each woman, her own concerns are of paramount importance. As such, rather than causing me existential pain, my wonderful patients provided me with solace. They taught me that each of us has a unique story. No matter how deep or shallow they may appear to others, none are more or less important. Unfortunately, the relationship with my patients did not help me with my needy young family. Sometimes I think that this preoccupation, along with my fatigue, may have actually made me less attentive to my husband and to my children.

As the old saying goes, I gave at the office.

Even to this day, there are nights that I cry myself to sleep.

I t was a beautiful Florida day in April 2003. The sky was clear, with a few scattered cumulous clouds softening an otherwise perfect blue canopy. It was warm but not hot, breezy but not windy. The humidity level was such that the skin felt supple, but the hair did not frizz. It was a day that reminded one why people chose to live in Florida. I drove to work and sat at my desk. I looked at the schedule. It was biopsy day. I had two stereotactic biopsies scheduled. These are procedures done on a patient with an abnormal mammographic finding. This minimally invasive procedure would identify the abnormality, and using computer localization, a relatively large bore needle would be inserted by me into the breast, a sample of tissue withdrawn and submitted for pathologic analysis. A Band-Aid would be applied, and the patient would go home that same day.

I rose from my desk and walked down the hall to the biopsy suite and walked inside. I looked around at the procedure room; machines with knobs, dials, numerical annotations, platforms, and breast compressors; infused with twinkling and fearsome medical sterility. I walked up to the patient—a forty-eight-year-old mother of three. She was a pretty brunette whose face, once a testimonial to society's definition of feminine pulchritude, was now etched with fine lines and tight lips—a silent smile that screamed her fears with deafening clarity. Looking directly into her beautiful dark eyes, I joyfully murmured my greeting, replete with soothing optimism and positive empathy while inwardly crying along with her in existential pain.

I walked back to the sterile tray. I looked at the equipment laid out on the sterile towel, gloves, prep swabs, gauze pads, syringes, needles, scalpels, small bottles of local anesthetic and saline, and a large bore biopsy needle. I glanced at the biopsy device or gun, the mammographic table, and the patient. Everything was prepared for performing a biopsy. I reminded myself. I performed these biopsies all the time. As I tried to effectively incorporate this into purposeful function, I felt a surreal, gentle but unwavering glove slip over my consciousness and cognition.

My technician, noting my hesitation, put on gloves and started to organize the equipment, softly muttering, "Here, Dr. Bachow..."

A few minutes passed before I regained full awareness. We were standing behind the chair in which my patient was seated. I walked around the chair, held her hand, and smiled. I gently told her that there was no problem with her but that I needed to transfer her to the hospital where the doctors there could perform the biopsy.

Unfortunately, I explained we had an equipment failure.

The medical assistant was summoned, and she took the patient out of the room to arrange for a transfer. There was then only the two of us. We were both silent for several minutes while I stared at the floor. My brain felt strangely empty. Eventually, my eyes found those of the technician. Instead of the earlier appearance of shock, hers were now softened with sadness. I'm sure she understood although she still had to ask...*equipment failure?* My throat tightened as my eyes started to fill. I raised my hand to my face, wiped off a mascara-laden tear, and slowly, painfully pointed my index finger at my head.

"Yes."

That night, I called my neurologist and explained what had happened. He listened closely and, in far more empathetic terms, said, "You're done."

I never saw another patient. My office was closed completely a few months later. I sold my practice to a local hospital and tearfully said goodbye to my staff, my office, referring physicians, and my thousands of patients. I also said goodbye to the person I was for years.

I spent countless hours learning about possible treatments. My neurologist described my illness as relapsing-progressive. Although my condition slowly and insidiously worsened, it was punctuated by temporary exacerbations, also called flares. These are short, often lasting hours to days, episodes of acute worsening of one or more symptoms, followed by regression of the symptom. Usually, after the resolution of the flare, the new baseline was a little worse than before.

As previously described in the review, relapsing-remitting MS is the most common variant in which MS flares would occur at varying frequencies but resolved nearly completely between episodes. The prescribed medical regimens are not designed to treat symptoms but instead are intended to minimize the number of flares. This is felt to delay advancement to the progressive form of the disease. Secondary-progressive MS is the one I had unfortunately developed, probably due to many years of unrecognized flares of RRMS. However, since I still experienced flares (and as the options available to treat the progressive disease were few, limited in both effectiveness and high risk for serious cardiac complications), I was initially treated with a variety of medications designed for relapsing-remitting MS, the more common, earlier form of the disease.

As I described earlier, my first injectable medication was administered subcutaneously (sub-Q), was given daily, and required refrigeration. There were almost no negative side effects except for reddening and some scarring at the injection sites. However, I could not discern any positive effects, so I stopped taking it. Looking back, I don't know why I expected to see an effect. The function of these drugs, or disease-modifying agents, is to minimize flares or relapses and, by doing so, slow down the natural progression of the disease. In other words, its desired effect was to make something not happen—a rather difficult concept to internalize. I then switched to one of the injectable interferons. These are man-made versions of a naturally occurring chemical in the body that controls the activity of the immune system. These interferons are supposed to reduce the frequency of exacerbations and stabilize the course of the disease.

It made sense to me.

As MS is a disease of an immune system going awry and attacking the patient's own cells (an *autoimmune* disease), treating it with interferons was a logical concept. I had to give myself *sub-Q* injections of this medication three times per week. Unfortunately, a side effect of this medication were severe flu-like symptoms, which for me lasted about forty-eight hours. In other words, I felt very ill from Monday through Friday. The symptoms started to abate over the weekend when I didn't inject interferons. On the weekend, Saturday daytime was hellish, Saturday night was tolerable, and Sunday was good. So every week, out of a total of 168 hours, I felt okay for about thirty-six hours. I felt awful for the remaining 132. But...who knows? Maybe it was slowing the progression of the disease? Maybe not? Meanwhile, for 132 hours a week, the side effects seemed worse than the disease. For me, this treatment didn't last long.

So I stopped everything. Bad decision. I became a patient rather than a physician and not a very intelligent patient, at that. I made decisions based upon anxiety, pain, discomfort, and denial... basically human emotions and fears rather than science and reason. But my local neurologist was okay with my decision. Apparently, he believed that I was destined to be wheelchair-bound shortly and likely to be bed-ridden before long...no matter what I did.

I continued on my slow downward spiral. You know, most people think of MS as a condition that interferes with the ability to walk. But it is so much more than this and more than numbness and tingling. It affects everything. Even the ability to think clearly and to be forgetful far beyond the scope of a senior moment. Even more surprising, one often loses control of emotions and the ability to respond to circumstances with the appropriate affect. For example, I might laugh when someone tells me something sad. People would be shocked and angry. Even I would be shocked and angry about what came out of my mouth.

This would tend to make one even more of a social outcast.

Wetting your pants without warning is not a particularly socially acceptable activity, either. Peeing down your leg in the aisle with pooling on the floor is frowned upon at Bloomingdales, even if you are a customer with a highly esteemed Bloomingdale's Black credit card.

After a short time, I progressed from a limp to a cane to a walker and was well on my way to a wheelchair. My local doctor seemed to be okay with that. I was slipping into advanced disability. Although the inability to walk was a significant motivating factor, it was the worsening of my other, more invisible symptoms which made me the most miserable. Being unable to walk is awful, but for me, it was not as unbearable as my loss of physiologic control of my body functions.

The recurrent bacterial urinary infections were often resistant to multiple antibiotics. Even when the infections were brought under control, they would cause a flare of my other MS symptoms. I missed the ability to regulate my emotions, and the progressive degree of cognitive decline was becoming more evident by the week. I would joke that of all the things I've lost in life, I miss my mind the most. But it wasn't really a joke. And severe fatigue, the fatigue could not be resolved by anything. And it made dealing with any other symptoms nearly impossible.

My Florida neurologist had discontinued all disease-modifying medications because of the intolerable side effects I had experienced with the several initial treatments I had tried. He basically threw up his hands and told me I would soon be wheelchair-bound.

I decided that it was time to do something.

My husband and I were from the northeast. The doctors who trained us in medical school, residency, and fellowship were in Massachusetts, Pennsylvania, and New York. Right or wrong, it was kind of like going home to our professional parents. So I started looking for specialists out of town.

Initially, I saw doctors in Massachusetts who were affiliated with Harvard Medical School. The first was a young but renowned doctor. Unfortunately, a few months after I became his patient, he decided to leave clinical practice and become employed by a pharmaceutical company involved in multiple sclerosis drug research. It's hard for me to blame him. I imagine this was both intellectually and financially rewarding.

The second was a very nice and renowned doctor in Cambridge, Massachusetts, who was recommended by a former professor with whom we were friendly.

This neurologist was very knowledgeable, understanding, and empathetic. In addition, she appeared to have mastery of the most recent research and recommendations. I thought I had found the answer to my dilemma, although I guess it was too good to be true.

After a short time, I was notified that the doctor had been seriously injured in an accident and could no longer care for patients. I was very sad for this lovely woman's misfortune. I am embarrassed to say that I was even sadder for my own.

So then I was off to the Big Apple.

There was a renowned multiple sclerosis specialist at one of the prominent New York City medical school university hospitals with whom I was fortunate enough to get an appointment. I'm embarrassed to say that this was one of the many advantages I had as a doctor. After multiple telephone calls, I was able to get an appointment. Unfortunately, it was for a few months later; however, apparently, I was lucky to get an appointment that year.

The time had finally come. My husband took time off from work, we found supervisory arrangements for our teenagers at home, and we embarked upon our journey, anticipating expert evaluation and recommendations from the guru.

Our flight to LaGuardia was delayed for no apparent reason, but as it was just a few years after 2001, delays of flights to New York were accepted without question. We had reservations in a three- to four-star hotel with decent online reviews and found ourselves in a room about the size of a South Florida master bath, which apparently is standard for Manhattan and not indicative of low-end lodging. Fortunately, my walker could fit in the room if I folded it and my husband carried it in sideways.

The next morning, we hailed a taxi, loaded my walker into the trunk of the cab and, full of palpable anticipation of a medical miracle, headed to the famous hospital to see the renowned specialist in search of the holy grail. Although there was nobody else in the waiting room, we sat there for about ninety minutes, thumbing through six-month-old *People* magazines.

After about one hour, my husband sheepishly went to the reception desk to check on the schedule, and with an odd combination of annoyance and boredom, the receptionist did not respond to his question but instead patronizingly hissed, "Please, sir. Be patient." She turned her supercilious glance toward me. "Barbara, is that your name?" she snarled. "PLEASE, Barbara, just wait until your name is called."

My husband's large eyes caught mine and were filled with bewildered sadness. This receptionist did not know or care who we were, more specifically, who I was. This unpleasant young woman was belittling me with her strong Brooklyn accent, which, sadly, was the beloved accent of my childhood. When I had first made the appointment, I told them I was a doctor. I didn't realize that I was just an out-of-town community doctor dwelling far removed from the ivory tower. Given my lowly pedigree, I was not granted any special professional status. In other words, here I was, an ordinary patient and was to be treated the way an ordinary patient was to be treated. It made me very sad. I was seeing a famous professor who taught residents. I didn't think that this was a way that I ever treated *my* patients.

Finally, my name was called, and I was escorted into the doctor's consulting room. The doctor was on the phone. He looked up at us and signaled with his hand toward the chairs across the desk from where he was seated, all while continuing his animated telephone conversation. I'm not entirely sure, but given the content of his speech and the agitation in his voice, I believe it was a personal call and likely with some sort of financial adviser. I actually was embarrassed for him. After about ten minutes, he hung up the phone, and while picking up my chart (and not maintaining eye contact), he began to speak.

"Barbara Bachow? And you were referred by…?"

The phone rang again. I expected him to buzz his secretary and request that his calls be held while he was consulting with a new patient…but he did not. It was another five minutes of agitated conversation. He seemed to be in a terrible mood.

"Self-referred?" He seemed almost angry with me!

"Why are you on no disease-modifying drugs?" As though it was my fault, his eyes were accusatory.

"My neurologist just stopped them after I found the side effects of the treatments he tried intolerable. He figured I would just progress eventually and at least be in a wheelchair before long." I was embarrassed as the words left my mouth. It was my fault. The New York specialist had me sit in a chair and, in silence, did a cursory neurological examination. He began to rattle off therapeutic options that my neurologist hadn't yet considered. He pointed out that my disease was progressive, which limited the efficacy of treatment options, but it was mandatory that I do something.

He did not give a specific treatment plan or offer to care for me himself. He just issued a consultation report to my Florida neurologist, which, in more eloquent terms, said that both my neurologist and I were stupid. Well, okay…not exactly. His telephone rang again, and he began another heated financial discussion. He waved us out, and we went to the front desk to sign out. My husband and I took an airline flight home the next day. We were both shaken.

This entire experience turned out to be one of many that, since my diagnosis, has filled me with both indignation and ignominy. To put it more simply, I was both angered and ashamed. The doctor was right, of course. But the way he treated me, in fact, the way he treated both of us, was both unsettling and upsetting. I guess I was learning how it felt to be sitting on the other side of the physician's desk and how it felt to be diminished in value and dehumanized by the doctor's attitude. In other words, how it felt to be a patient. I prayed that I had actually never treated my patients like that.

Upon my return home, I made an appointment to see my local Florida neurologist. I sat silently as he read the report from the New York specialist, turning the pages very slowly and staring down at the typed pages. He slowly stroked his gray-thinning hair and shifted his gaze upon me briefly, his face virtually expressionless except for one eyebrow locked in a raised position, horizontal lips, and a glazed stare. He was obviously pissed off. He pulled down the roll of white waxy paper, sat me on the examination table, and performed a cursory neurological exam in complete silence. He picked up a pen and a pad and wrote a prescription for another common disease-modifying drug. This was one I had not yet been treated with; however, it was another interferon drug, and therefore similar to the one I could not tolerate before.

With no further discussion, he was simply responding to the insulting consultation and, therefore, did something. His office staff called in the prescription. I left the office in silence. The entire experience was awful. And once again, so was the treatment.

I vowed to keep searching for the doctor who could help me, one who could improve my current symptoms, and who could somehow change the rate of symptomatic decline. Like every other sufferer with multiple sclerosis (and yes…like many with no real medical knowledge), I was looking for a miracle worker.

My sister-in-law (my husband's sister) was an affluent New Yorker who, at the time, was living on the Upper East Side of Manhattan. She and her husband were professionally affiliated with another financially successful banker who, incidentally, suffered with multiple sclerosis. Given his influential position in the world of high finance, he had connections that enabled him to establish substantial fundraisers for causes he deemed worthy. His neurologist, a renowned multiple sclerosis specialist, had left his university medical school affiliation to establish a center devoted to both patient care as well as innovative research into the cause, diagnosis, treatment, and potential cure of multiple sclerosis. This doctor understood that although patients diagnosed with MS shared an underlying condition with similar basic pathophysiology, the mechanics of each patient's disease is their own and is ladened with variability, each requiring an individualized (and often evolving) therapy. In the long term, the doctor's research would offer insight into the possible causes and potential cures for MS. In the short term, it offered innovative, creative, and specialized therapeutic plans designed exclusively for each patient.

These were lofty and costly goals. The doctor required ongoing financial support for this investigative and clinical venture that went far beyond the scope of the typical research grants he had readily been granted. As one of his grateful patients, the investment banker established a fundraiser to support the doctor's foundation, and my sister-in-law and her husband (as another such banker) were invited as prospective donors. She and her husband made a sizable contribution.

You know, sometimes you just have to be lucky.

At last, I had found the right doctor. He evaluated me as a woman with multiple sclerosis, as a retired, disabled physician, and as a distinct, individual human being. We connected and began a journey into my present and future, both medically and personally. It would be truly wonderful if everyone with a chronic illness could be so fortunate.

I began treatment with less common regimens. My neurologist was in New York City, and I lived in South Florida, so arrangements for my local therapy were a bit more complicated than usual. After finally establishing *doctor-patient* relationships with local physicians, I was able to obtain intravenous medication on a regular schedule at their infusion centers by becoming a patient of theirs. Several of these doctors were actually oncologists (cancer doctors) but were appropriately trained to monitor my infusion therapy. I was then treated with various regimens, each for approximately two years and each with some efficacy. Efficacy, you might recall, was difficult to determine because, as I explained earlier, success was based upon something not happening. In any case, after about two years, I would be switched to another treatment, each with a similar course. The choice of therapy was difficult as nearly all treatment regimens were for the more common *relapsing-remitting* MS.

My diagnosis was a form of progressive MS, which is felt to be somewhat different, and for which no satisfactory protocol was available. (There was one infusion medication that might help but was associated with irreversible heart failure. No thanks.) I had occasional allergic reactions (occasionally serious), which were managed successfully.

And my multiple sclerosis progressed. Perhaps it progressed more slowly than it would have without treatment but who knew for sure. My fatigue was overwhelming. This is a common problem with MS. No amount of sleep would help. Nonetheless, I could never fall asleep.

My numbness and intermittent inability to move my limbs worsened. I fell frequently and occasionally had significant fractures, breaking my humerus in my right arm, requiring surgery with a titanium plate and screws, and a fall resulting in multiple pelvic fractures, necessitating a long period of rehabilitation. I developed frequent bouts of severe stabbing pain in my right face and ear (particularly at night), which was similar to a condition known as trigeminal neuralgia, nicknamed by medical professionals as the suicide disease—no further explanation needed.

I had to pee constantly and had limited control. There is nothing more embarrassing than peeing on the floor at Bloomingdales. And even so, I was not emptying my bladder adequately enough, so I had to begin bladder self-catheterization, or inserting a tube into my bladder, several times a day and allowing the urine to drain. This, of course, led to frequent urinary tract infections, which became increasingly more difficult to control. Not only were these painful, but since I was so frequently treated with antibiotics, I developed bacteria that were resistant to antibiotics, such that we needed to use the end-of-the-line antibiotics (beyond which there were essentially no more available) for treatment. I eventually developed pyelonephritis, which means my infection extended from my bladder to my kidney, which is far more serious. This required hospitalization and close follow-up by infectious-disease specialists. This specialist told me that from now on I should not present for treatment of urinary infections until I started peeing pus. She said that I should not be treated unless I developed back pain, which is a symptom of pyelonephritis, or kidney infection, which can progress to kidney failure, blood sepsis, and death. Her explanation was that I had reached the end game of antibiotics, and if I developed resistance to that drug, I was going to die. I was shocked and overwhelmed. Although what she said was obvious, I had never heard it articulated before.

I left her office and promptly had a car accident.

At this time, I need to make a confession. At some point, I slipped into a deep depression that lasted years. I did nothing and was essentially useless to myself and my family. I basically communicated with nobody. I would watch the news on television and play bubble-pop games on my smartphone all day. I rarely read anything, the least of which were medical journals. My husband ordered and picked up dinner. My eldest son had already left for college, so he wasn't affected. But my second son was in high school, and my baby daughter was in middle school. As do all children, they had issues that required motherly love and guidance. But I wasn't there.

They are five years apart in age but would talk to each other all the time. Dad was working all the time, and I was essentially absent. I guess they sought advice from each other. Often, their advice to each other was juvenile, inexperienced, and not the best, but they and their friends were their only options.

And living with me made them sad.

They are grown now and are wonderful, functional adults. But they missed out on a doting, involved mother during their adolescence. I cannot forgive myself. I'm sure that they, too, will never forget.

I guess their experiencing my illness had one positive side effect. As I recall, years ago, my thirteen-year-old daughter pushed me in a wheelchair while we walked in the mall. A former patient of mine approached us with her husband and began gushing and telling my daughter she loved me, I had saved her life, and that I was such a caring doctor.

As the woman walked away, I glanced at my daughter, who was rolling her eyes.

Another happy customer…, she muttered.

Years later, that little girl went to medical school, became a physician, and performed with unparalleled empathy. And her patients love her. Go figure.

As I slowly reentered life, I started to focus on helping myself. I began many uncommon treatments for progressive MS. One such treatment involves a spinal tap every six weeks with the instillation of chemotherapy. As with all my other treatments, this helped for a while. It was followed by three months of weekly transfusions of plasma, for which I had to temporarily move to New York City. When I returned home, I began intravenous infusion, administered by a home-health nurse every three weeks, of IVIG or other people's antibodies. I assume the idea was that these other antibodies would not attack my nerve cells like my own stupid antibodies. I underwent this therapy for five years.

During this time, I focused on my urinary issues. I decided I didn't want to die, certainly not from the nightmare of sepsis or blood poisoning due to an untreatable urinary tract infection.

So as the saying goes…doctor heal thyself.

Amazingly, after years of suffering, I decided to use my dormant understanding of medicine. I scientifically designed a technique that would dramatically reduce the number of urinary tract infections in a patient with my clinical issues. In fact, the few times that a bladder infection did occur, it was no longer caused by a bacterial strain resistant to standard antibiotics and could be treated easily without significant risk. Essentially, I saved my own life.

So that other patients with similar issues could benefit from my technique should their doctors recommend it, I wrote up my discovery as a case report which I submitted to a medical journal. To my amazement, it was published and appeared online. Doctors could read it and use the technique for the care of patients suffering with a similar therapeutic dilemma. Urologist friends of mine began recommending my technique to their patients.

I couldn't help but feel an indescribable joy. I am still a doctor. In an unusual way, I was back.

After five years, the frequent IVIG infusions started to become very rough on my veins, and I was getting close to the point of needing an in-dwelling chemotherapy port. The port offers a site of deep, intravenous access and is surgically inserted under the skin on the right side of the chest. It is then threaded into a large deep chest vein near the heart. This would provide ready, easy intravenous access without relying on my diminishing peripheral veins. It has the possibility of both early and late complications, but serious complications are relatively uncommon. In the clinical setting in which such a port is needed, it is felt to have a satisfactory risk/benefit ratio. I was ready.

But timing is everything.

It was then that my neurologist told me about a new drug that was different from the others in that it was specifically helpful in the treatment of progressive forms of multiple sclerosis, which is my diagnosis. Nearly all the disease-modifying drugs previously available were designed for the treatment of relapsing-remitting MS. Because there were essentially no good options, those of us with progressive forms of the disease were given those medications anyway. This new medication is an immunosuppressant that directly interferes with the cells in the body that create the antibodies that destroy nerve function. It directly interferes with the mechanism of action of multiple sclerosis. And even more amazingly, it is administered by intravenous infusion at a doctor's office twice a year. Having had almost twenty years of very frequent, life-controlling, invasive, uncomfortable, dangerous procedures in the past, I was eager to embark upon this new venture.

In 2021, I was administered my first COVID-19 vaccine. After several weeks, I had several blood tests and began my therapy. I am not sure if I am imagining it, but I believe my symptoms are dramatically improved. I feel better than I have in years.

I have often said that there is a particularly difficult aspect to being a physician with a chronic disease. When doctors talk to such patients, they emphasize the positive. They focus on what the patient can personally do to improve his or her condition, allowing the patient a chance to feel that they have some control over their illness. This is enormously helpful. By relieving the feeling of impotence, the patient not only feels better but actually medically does better, with improvement of their odds. I believe that achieving that in a patient is part of the art of practicing medicine.

The problem is that when you are a doctor, you are a creature of data and statistics. You cannot incorporate the intangible into your own experience. I have no doubt that it is extremely effective both emotionally and medically when dealing with patients, and I have seen this intangible advice genuinely improve outcomes. However, it is different for the doctor as a patient. Doctors are extensively educated in biology and pathophysiology. We are actually trained to think concretely, with a logical assessment of probabilities and statistics in the diagnosis and treatment of disease.

When talking to patients, as I described, we are working with the intangible. Seeking personal strengthening to feel power over disease was something that I found very effective, and patients often actually did better medically. No matter the outcome, at least they felt better. Unfortunately, the intangible does not work for a doctor when they are the patient. As I have said, I read the book.

But there was actually no intangible here. I was feeling better. I believe I will be on this medication for more than my usual two years. I can now walk either unassisted or with a walker, and when going significant distances with my husband, I take my walker that has a reversible strap and retractable footrests such that it can readily be converted from a walker to a wheelchair. Therefore, when I get too tired to walk, we can convert the walker and continue the stroll as my husband pushes me in the chair.

Last week, we went for a long walk in a local park. There was lush Everglades vegetation and many noisy tropical birds. We were debating whether these were egrets or herons (although, in fact, they may very well have been neither). An older couple approached us. The woman gently touched my arm.

"Dr. Bachow?"

I turned and faced her. I saw a seventyish-year-old woman with graying hair and soft features. She was a pretty older lady. She told me her name.

I must admit that with nine thousand patients, I did not remember each one. When I ran into patients outside the office and did not remember who they were, I would explain that with so many patients, I would clearly remember those with a difficult, complicated evaluation or a serious problem. They were then happy to know I didn't remember them.

I remembered this lady.

She saw me annually from age forty-five. When she was about fifty, she developed a subtle but suspicious finding. I performed a biopsy, and she had very small but aggressive breast cancer. I referred her to a surgeon, and she began a long but successful course of therapy. The surgeon actually called me to say that the mammographic finding was so subtle that he had discussed it with the patient. He told me that she had thanked him for saving her life. He apparently told her that he was just part of the process and that, in fact, "Dr. Bachow saved your life."

Shortly after this diagnosis, I retired because of my illness and did not see the patient in follow-up.

Now about twenty years later, here she was. When I looked up at the couple, the husband was smiling, with tears running down his cheeks.

The woman gazed at me and said, "I don't know how I can ever thank you."

She then looked at my husband behind the wheelchair and, with joy on her face, proclaimed, "And you must be married to Dr. Bachow!"

I turned quickly to look at my husband's face. Married to Dr. Bachow? My husband was Dr. Bachow for well over forty years. In fact, he was Dr. Bachow before I was Dr. Bachow, and he was still practicing medicine. He was still a real Dr. Bachow. Approximately ten seconds passed, although it felt like time was standing still. I looked at my husband's face. It was older, but he still had those large blue eyes, albeit now rimmed laterally with crow's feet. They had an unmistakable look of bewilderment at the woman's question. His lips were held tight and straight, and I felt a nervous twitch in my own face as I looked at him. A few seconds later, I could see his eyes soften. Then slowly, one corner of his mouth crept upward into that youthful, lopsided grin we had shared years before.

"Married to Dr. Bachow?" He put his hand on my shoulder. He looked into the woman's eyes and said, "Am I married to Dr. Bachow?" His eyes caught mine as he proclaimed, "Yes, I am!"

The End

ABOUT THE AUTHOR

Dr. Bachow graduated from Cornell University and received her MD from the University of Massachusetts Medical School.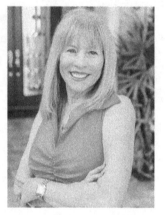

She trained in Internal Medicine at Tufts Medical Center and completed a residency in Diagnostic Radiology at Beth Israel Hospital in Boston, where she was a clinical fellow at Harvard Medical School. She was certified by the American Board of Radiology in 1984.

She began to practice general diagnostic radiology in South Florida in 1985, eventually opening the Center for Mammography and Breast Diagnostics in Deerfield Beach, Florida. The center was dedicated to the clinical and radiological diagnosis of breast disease.

The practice was remarkably successful.

During her practice, she served as chairman of the Breast Cancer Task Force of the Florida Division of the American Cancer Society. She was honored by the Weizmann Institute as a *woman of vision*.

Then in 2003, it was all over.

Printed in the USA
CPSIA information can be obtained
at www.ICGtesting.com
LVHW091542221024
794497LV00002B/340

9 798889 823957